Also by June Goodfield

COURIER TO PEKING
THE GROWTH OF SCIENTIFIC PHYSIOLOGY

Co-Author
THE FABRIC OF THE HEAVENS
THE ARCHITECTURE OF MATTER
THE DISCOVERY OF TIME

the
SIEGE
of
CANCER

the
SIEGE
of
CANCER

G. JUNE GOODFIELD

RANDOM HOUSE 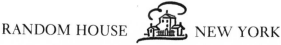 NEW YORK

Grateful acknowledgment is made to the following for permission to reprint
previously published material:

American Association for the Advancement of Science and Drs. Mead and
Métraux: For the article "Image of the Scientist Among High-School Students"
by Margaret Mead and Rhoda Métraux. Reprinted from *Science*, Vol. 126,
pages 384–390, August 30, 1957.

American Medical Association and Gail McBride: For excerpts from her article
entitled "The Sloan-Kettering affair: Could it have happened anywhere?" from
The Journal of the American Medical Association, Vol. 229, No. 11, pages
1391–1410. Copyright © 1974 by the American Medical Association.

Harcourt Brace Jovanovich, Inc.: For six lines from Act II, Scene iii of *The
Family Reunion* by T. S. Eliot. Copyright 1939 by T. S. Eliot, renewed 1967 by
Esme Valerie Eliot.

Library of Congress Cataloging in Publication Data
Goodfield, G June.
The siege of cancer.
1. Cancer. I. Title. [DNLM: 1. Neoplasms—
Popular works. QZ201 G651s]
RC262.G64   616.9'94'0072   75-10298
ISBN 0-394-49119-X

9 8 7 6 5 4 3 2

First Edition

For
Charlotte and Martin Goodfield
and to the memory of
David,
their father, my brother.

*"Far better 'tis to die
the death that flashes gladness,
than alone, in frigid dignity,
to live on high.
Better, in burning sacrifice
be thrown against the world
to perish, than the sky
to circle endlessly
a barren stone."*

The Shooting Star; author unknown.
Quoted in Nature, August 26, 1933.

PREFACE

In a very real sense only a small part of this book comes from my mind and my pen. For in writing about the people with cancer and those who study cancer, I have depended almost totally on their ideas, work, experience and feelings. Except in the case of two friends who, with their doctors, admitted me into the private world of suffering and decision, I have used real names throughout. All the scientists who figure strongly in this book have read it in manuscript, and their comments have been most helpful in maintaining its scientific accuracy. Where errors occur this is my responsibility alone. But if their critical advice has been helpful, their forbearance has been remarkable. So too has been their willingness to go with me through a process of personal and scientific assessment. I only hope that something of my gratitude and deep affection emerges from these pages.

Several things must be stressed. First, though I did not select the scientists and institutions I chose to study by an entirely random process, this choice should in no way be interpreted as a sure index of crucial discoveries in cancer. At this stage it is quite impossible to decide where breakthroughs will come: all I can do is present a cross section of people and research. So while some people will undoubtedly feel irritated that the obviously brilliant work of Dr. X in Institute Y has been omitted, I must emphasize that I never tried either to cover all cancer research or to wear the mantle of a prophet. I have focused on five main areas within contemporary work, but even within these, I have concentrated on one or two individuals only, trying to see the problems through their eyes. Second, though I studied the problem of cancer and viruses mostly at the Sloan-Kettering Institute for Cancer Research in New York, and cancer and the immune system at University College, London, it could easily have been the other way around, for nearly all places and subjects were interchangeable. Had I chosen any other place, or inverted the situations, only the people, their personalities and the detailed problems would have been different. The general conclusions about the state of the art would have been identical. Third, my emphasis is more on the American scene than on the rest of the world; I apologize to those who may be hurt, but there is an inevitability about it. America has made a conscious decision to invest heavily in cancer research, and in proportion, a greater amount of work is being done there. So if Chapter 6, which discusses the politics of research, concentrates almost exclusively on the problems that arise within the American context, this is because only there is the level of support so great as to generate these problems.

I have, of course, incurred debts to many other people whom I have never met: to the thousands around the world whose work, too, adds to the sum of our present knowledge about cancer; to reporters and writers of articles in such journals as *Nature* and *Scientific American.* I am especially grateful to Barbara Culliton and Thomas Maugh II, staff writers for *Science,* whose words have been most helpful signposts over the last two years. More formally, I want to thank the various institutions who gave me facilities and help: The Institute of

Public Health of Iran; The Sloan-Kettering Institute for Cancer Research, New York; The Chester Beatty Insitute, London; University College, London.

But I owe a very special debt indeed, both personal and professional, to the dean and faculty of the College of Human Medicine, Michigan State University. Friends and colleagues, they have for some years now warmly included me into many aspects of their work and lives. I have learned enormously from them in a whole variety of ways, and so far as I am concerned their influence is stamped on every page of this book.

Finally I must thank those who were close to me throughout the research and writing: Hilary Rubinstein, Gerard McCauley and Francis Bennett of Hutchinson, who with encouragement, enthusiasm and sometimes admonition helped me develop what writing talents I possess; Jim Silberman and Neil Nyren of Random House, whose salutary and painful editorial advice at a critical stage in the writing launched us immediately into a love-hate relationship of great value; Joan Thornton, always willing to be interrupted and always ready with perceptive and loving comments; Ann Wickens and Julie Eastman, who type beautiful manuscripts. Above all, I owe a great debt to Joy Cull, who has sustained me in innumerable ways these last years, providing skilled help and a constant encouragement which never wilts, though I do sometimes. So one day, when in a mood of pessimistic fatigue I said, "I don't think I can write this book," she replied, "Oh, but you can," with such quiet conviction that there was nothing else for it except to pick up my pen and continue.

—June Goodfield

Since Chapters 3, 4 and 5 inevitably contain some technicalities, a short glossary has been provided at the end of this book.

CONTENTS

the
SIEGE
of
CANCER

PROLOGUE

CANCER TOUCHES US ALL

The young man, or woman, writing today has forgotten the problems of the human heart in conflict with itself, which alone can make good writing, because only that is worth writing about, worth the agony and the sweat.

—William Faulkner, from his
speech accepting the Nobel
Prize for Literature

The Real Inspector Hound, by Tom Stoppard, is quite literally a play within a play. The entire action revolves around two drama critics seated next to the stage, which is furnished as a drawing room. At one key moment the stage is empty and a telephone begins to ring. No one comes to answer it. Finally, one of the critics can stand it no longer. He runs onto the stage, picks up the receiver, and listens. Then he turns to the other man and says, "It's for you." His colleague leaves his seat and comes down to take the call, but as he is speaking one of the characters comes onto the stage. At this point, the stage directions read, "Everything is as it was. It is, let us say, the same moment of time." For the critic, however, time has moved on and it is too late. He is caught up in the action and plays out the play with the others, unable ever to withdraw.

This is what it has been like these last two years. I came to this work in a state of acute sensitivity, with feelings raw and emotions heightened by a series of unexpected personal blows.

A small rent had appeared in the fabric of my life and widened with such speed that suddenly I was left holding the shreds of my past in my hands, with no way of ever patching it together again. So when Hilary, who for some years now has gently steered me through my writing, suggested that the time was ripe for a new book about cancer, I welcomed the opportunity. It was a good suggestion and seemed a safe one, safe because in my ragged state the experience would provide a temporary haven. I could work on an objective, dispassionate account of the most difficult problem in biology, topped off by a judicious appraisal of the problem and state of the art, and the storms of feelings would pass me by.

I was very simple-minded, with a naïveté that I can now only attribute to the amnesia that finally enters memory and dulls the edge of grief. But the naïveté did not last long. For then David, my brother, died, plucked quietly out of life one warm spring afternoon. It was not from cancer but a stroke due to a small defect in the wall of a blood vessel, in all probability present from the day he was born. So in unconscious ignorance he slipped gently into the darkness, and death reminded me that it provides the only permitted withdrawal from life.

I had been with him and his family the very day before. With friends I was passing through Petersfield on the way to the boat that would take us to the Iberian Peninsula for a vacation. So it was not till four days later that Joy finally reached me on the telephone. The details of memory are etched with a fine pen at such moments. I remember protesting in an utter and total disbelief, resisting the news for some three hours till the reality finally penetrated; then, shivering with shock, I entered a second and separate year of grief. The total, irrevocable fact that lay with me that night was the single event that finally knocked me out of a state of intellectual arrogance and absorbed withdrawal. Death is immediate and death is real.

So now I find my previous blithe state of objectivity quite appalling. For cancer is *not* an intellectual problem. It begins and ends with people, some who live and some who die, some who suffer and some who try to cure the suffering. This book is about them all, but especially about the doctors and scientists who are trying to understand cancer. If I wanted to write about any of them I would have to become involved, be caught up in the action and play out the play.

To begin, I watched two separate stages. One was a scientific stage where the central theme was the analysis and solution of an intellectual problem, and its solution would mean not only an understanding of a puzzle, but its therapeutic application to the world of patients. On the second stage the experience was more immediate and everything was interpreted in terms of people's feelings and lives, whether doctors or patients. Many people and many experiences provided the links between the two stages. If I was ever tempted to concentrate on one theme to the exclusion of the other, a person or an event would pull me back. It was Bernie Horner who did so most consistently. Bernie is one of the drivers at the Sloan-Kettering Institute for Cancer Research, and several times a day he drives the station wagon between the laboratories in Manhattan and the laboratories out at Rye, transporting people, mail, specimens and equipment. At one point I was taking the wagon every day, riding during the quiet midmorning period. One morning we began to talk about cancer. Two evenings before Bernie had seen a television documentary program on cancer, *The Killers*. It had made a great impact. "You know," he said, "I've seen 'it.' I asked Linda, one of the technicians, to show me the 'cancer' cell, and she did. I ask you, how could anything so small be so damaging, so deadly? I've seen the people too," Bernie went on. "That cancer therapy, it's a rough ride. One woman on the program said that the treatment was worse than the disease, and it was. Then I see people all around, griping, yelling their heads off for more money or something. They take their health for granted. They don't know that they've got the most important thing. I tell you," he concluded, "it shook me up."

It shook me up, too—not so much illness, death and dying, or illness, cure and life, for I saw all these in cancer. What shook me up was being brought face to face with human suffering, in situations of uncertainty. There is a limbo state about cancer that makes it one of the most difficult problems to cope with. The chances now of living, and living well, are so much higher than they were ten years ago, yet at the back of one's mind there must always be—as Stewart Alsop said in his book *Stay of*

Execution—"the little pea of fear . . . the fear of death . . . always present like a kind of background music." It was because of this, I think, that I reacted with a small spurt of cold anger to a flip young American whom I met at the American Institute in Tehran. On hearing that I had been up to study the work going on amongst the Turkoman tribes, he said, dismissively, "We have more important problems in the world than cancer." No doubt he meant it seriously, even though he didn't specify these problems, but I believe only someone who regarded cancer as an intellectual problem alone could have spoken like this. Now, through David, Bernie, Jan and Rachel, I am not likely to forget that the climax of all the work I saw will be the alleviation—if possible, the prevention—of a condition which affected me deeply. It affected me most of all in Rachel and Jan, whose stories I tell in the last chapter.

Rachel I saw first in a hospital bed. She had been admitted only two days before with a severe throat infection. Twenty-four hours before, she had been told she had acute leukaemia. When I first went into her room, I was not with her physician, nor her cancer specialist, nor even the haematologist, all of whom were to give her—and continue to give her—such devoted care. I was one of a small group, a couple of medical students taken on rounds by yet another specialist and a young intern. Later her doctor was to say that when you tell patients they have acute leukaemia, you may talk for fifteen to twenty minutes, trying to explain, but they will only have heard those two words. For they are trying to take in the phrase and all it means. By the time we saw Rachel the meaning had just begun to penetrate, for she was talking with the specialist with only half her mind focused, and I heard the discussion with only half my mind, too. There was no doubt we were all aware of what we were doing. Possibly no one can be blamed, but outside her door the specialist said he knew she wanted to cry with someone at that moment, but "Right now we don't have time." The human element was ignored, and as a group we walked out.

Jan came to see me of his own accord. He telephoned my office one day and came up in his car to take me back to his home for lunch. There could be no mistaking him—the long, taut face, with the skin drawn tight over his head. It was clear that the cancer was getting right to him. He looked very tired, but as our talk progressed he rallied. We went back to his home, sat in the sun outside the drawing room, made lunch and talked. He has had much personal tragedy in his life, culminating in the death of his son, so this makes cancer for him, "not a big thing, just one more mutilation." He was struggling with so much: with his illness; with the limbo that cancer inflicts, because there is nothing inevitable about it and there is always hope; with the pain; with the slow erosion of health; with the knowledge of his family's distress; and with a practical situation that I felt was an intolerable and uncalled-for burden. Somehow he had to live another three months, for then the insurance would take care of his wife and children. As if to mute the demands of mortality, he was struggling hard at the same time to do something for others, organizing a group, preparing papers for people who may one day be in his situation, telling them what may be involved, telling them where they can turn for help, both practical and medical. He came to see me, however, because he wanted to talk about death and dying.

With Rachel and Jan, I felt impotent and distressed. Yet this was an experience I would not have missed, for through it I learned so much, matured with them and understood things that I had never known before. Here the two actions merge, for these human lives represent the backdrop, permanent in its presence, changing in its detail, against which the drama of the scientific work will always be played.

Talking one evening to a most perceptive and sensitive physician about the frustrations and successes, agonies and exultations that arise with cancer, I was given a wise injunction to serve both me and everyone else. "Above all, you must not think you can play God," he warned me. "It is enough just to be human."

But the temptation to play God is very real, and so is the equally dangerous wish to seek miracles where none may be legitimately expected. We are not many years away from the times when men used to ascribe godlike powers to doctors and even to scientists. As the first nuclear explosion flashed into the morning sky, Robert Oppenheimer was to recall the lines of Sri Krishna, the Exalted One: "I am become Death, the shatterer of worlds"; others, on smaller occasions, have seen the problem of cancer as demanding similar powers. In 1911, when Henry James was sixty-eight, he was taken on a tour of the Rockefeller University by Simon Flexner, the director. He visited the laboratory of Dr. Peyton Rous, who at the age of thirty-three was on the verge of his discovery about the relationship between viruses and cancer. Dr. Flexner introduced him as the man in charge of cancer research. Forthwith, according to Rous, "Mr. James clapped a heavy hand on my shoulder, and exclaimed in a resounding voice, 'How magnificent! To be young and have divine power!' " Faced with a situation of which he knew very little, James in his paternalistic way was trying to do his best for the young man, make him feel at ease, but Rous was so flustered that he tacitly acknowledged the divinity, answering only that he was not as young as he looked!

We know better now than to seek divinity from scientists, and scientists know better than to make such claims. Knowledge, not divinity, will enable us to solve the intellectual side of the problem, and the need for scientific knowledge as a basis for medicine has been recognized for some time. Nearly one hundred years ago, in 1887, T. H. Huxley was asked to address the International Medical Congress in London. As usual, he had some pithy things to say about the state of medical knowledge:

> Even the practising physician, while nowise underestimating the regulative value of accurate diagnosis, must often lament that so much of his knowledge rather prevents him from doing wrong than helps him to do right. A scorner of physic once said that nature and disease may be compared to two men fighting, the doctor to a blind man with a club, who strikes into the mêlée, sometimes hitting the disease, and sometimes hitting nature . . . He had better not meddle at all until his eyes are opened—until he can see the exact position of the antagonists, and make sure of his blows.

Huxley pleaded for a far greater study of physiology and biology in medicine so that we might eventually come to see disease with clear vision. A proper understanding of the biology would give us a proper basis for therapy. The image of doctors as blind men with clubs is true only in parts of our present-day medicine, but even so, when we consider cancer as a biological problem, we are only just a little further along than the ancient doctors of Egypt and Greece who first recorded the symptoms and the various kinds of treatment. For centuries man has known cancer as a human disease. For decades biologists have known cancer as grotesque alterations in organisms from gingko trees to fruit flies to lobsters and man. But as we come to know cancer, we realize how complicated it is, for much more is involved than just a normal cell turning into an abnormal one. Cancer is an amalgam of several sorts of diseases involving the whole organism. We are faced not only with the pathological condition of a given organ but with the interplay of every system in the whole body. Even so, scientists now do not believe that cancer is all that much more complicated than many other forms of chronic disease which occur late in life—rheumatism, arthritis or auto-immune disease may be even more difficult to cure. But with cancer we are dealing with two levels of complexity all the time. On the one hand, there is the intellectually challenging concept of the most difficult theoretical problems in biology. What is it that makes a normal cell transform into a malignant one? What makes it fail to respond to normal growth-controlling stimuli? What is it that makes a cell slip away and spread in the insidious process of cancer metastasis? Superimposed on this, however, is the additional massive complexity which comes when the organs of the body interact with other disease-fighting mechanisms, such as the hormones and the immune-defense system. So in dealing with a malignant cell, we have both the first cellular event and its growth, and then the spread of the cancer throughout the whole organism. T. H. Huxley's doctor, that blind man with his club, can consider himself a man of sight only when he understands everything that is going on during the entire series of events.

Yet in one sense we have not known cancer at all, even after all this time. Our attitude toward the disease has never been entirely rational. Throughout history it has been a hopeless challenge to doctors, a baffling riddle to scientists, and until quite recently, a death sentence to patients. Each group in its own way acquired its own particular fatalism or fear. Sir Richard Doll, Regis Professor of Medicine at Oxford and a world authority on lung cancer and epidemiology, recalls a colleague of his, a professor of surgery, who even as late as the 1940's stated flatly that it was not only a waste of time, but even immoral to try to prevent cancer. He was expressing in an extreme form the degree of pessimism which predominated only twenty years ago. Medically and scientifically, the problem was one of the most appalling complexity, and there seemed little that could be done to reduce cancer mortality, let alone prevent the disease. Sir Peter Medawar has written of the despondent air in cancer institutes in the thirties, the moroseness derived from a "very well-founded sense of inadequacy" when their efforts were set against the magnitude of the problem. Cancer was the great failure of medicine—an accusation often heard, reflecting the bitterness of public opinion in the face of impotence and defeat.

Even the very name was disquieting. The Greeks brought the word into our language; Galen, a famous Greek physician, tells us that tumors were given this name because the surrounding veins become distended with pressure and look like the limbs of a crab. Though Galen's interpretation may have been very matter-of-fact, others have wondered whether Hippocrates chose the name because of the clawing pain and constant, steady growth. The image of something eating away at one's very substance is the image of fear with which people have lived. The stealthiness, the irrevocableness, the pain, the hopelessness at the sight of those people who seem dead and forgotten among the living—all in turn have contributed to an edifice of fear, irrationality and ignorance. Modern investigators, looking at the cultural and social context of cancer, have described our attitudes as a "kind of cultural fear—a hard instinct, rooted in prejudice and ignorance, containing moral, magical and retributive elements." For years statistics carried false entries made in deference to the wishes of relatives, who felt about the word "cancer" as they did about "suicide" and did not wish that cause of death to appear in the records.

Cancer may not be the number one killer, but it is the one that people still fear most, and there is a reason for this. Of the two hundred million Americans alive in 1975, fifty-three million will develop cancer—that is, over a quarter of the population—and one in six of all deaths will be from cancer. In the face of such facts, it is not surprising that faith in science and medicine breaks down, that ignorance becomes our refuge, and quackery as much as medicine becomes our defense.

Recalling Richard Doll's sceptical professor, we see that faith in medicine broke down even among the people who were practicing it. But now, thirty years later, one senses the quickening pulse of optimism, and sees the emergence of a new confidence. Just why this exists and on just what it is based was one of the things I set out to find, trying to catch the present state of the art. This new exhilaration comes not because there have been striking breakthroughs, but because, once again, using well-tried methods of science we finally see that this problem can also be made to yield, and in certain areas is already breaking. For those men and women with whom I was to live for nine months, the climax of their work, their victory, will be not merely the confirming of an idea or the establishment of a theory, but the solution of a human problem which, when it comes, will blur again the false distinction between science, technology and the human art. For medicine humanely applied is all these things.

It is in a mood of optimistic ignorance, motivated by a desire to understand and a desire to help, that scientists are now approaching the problem of cancer, and it was in this same mood that I went to find them. What I tried to cover was a genuine cross section of human effort. Some twenty or thirty people were selected from tens of thousands of scientists in some four or five institutions from the ten or so really prestigious centers of cancer research in the whole world. I came to be with these people partly by historical accident, partly through friends, partly by reading about intriguing research, then finally by being handed on from scientist to scientist as the work progressed.

The pages of this book are studded with neither the gems of Nobel laureates nor those of scientists who make certain that they make the headlines. The former genuinely do trail clouds of glory; the latter, more often than not, trail vapor. But I cannot tell yet where the real successes in cancer research will come, nor, I suspect, can anyone else, though scientists armed with the weapons of knowledge, prejudice and informed hunch may be able to make a more realistic appraisal.

Certainly some of the people in these pages *will* achieve striking scientific success, and possibly the glittering rewards that follow. But however gratifying the scientific crown, the real significance of the work lies elsewhere. It will affect Rachel's life, Jan's life, everyone's life. For ultimately cancer touches us all; if only because we have had it or known friends with it, or because we have shared fears about it, or most importantly, because it is a human problem and we are all human beings together.

I began first in Iran.

1

CANCER AND OUR WORLD:
BUT DO THE HORSES GET IT?

THE FILE LAY on the table between us, a mute, uncomplaining witness. It bore my name and, to my complete bewilderment, the stamp *Highly Confidential.* Inside were the letters that, a year earlier, I had churned out in duplicate and triplicate requesting permission to visit the research teams working on oesophageal cancer in an area northeast of the Caspian Sea. It was very mild stuff, indeed: my vitae, various reprints, the details of what I wished to study, and covering letters of recommendation from the dean and the chairman of my department in Michigan, Andy Hunt and Bill Callaghan. Everything was set out in precise detail, following a bureaucratic formula recommended by friends in Tehran.

There was silence around the table. We lifted our glasses in turn and drank the tea that is served in Iran on every occasion, formal or informal. Audrey Lambert, whose exemplary diplomatic skill had finally brought me together with these people, was smiling gently as she waited for the moment when she could properly leave us and return to the hundred and one pinpricks of a British Council representative in a capital city. I looked across at Dr. Janez Kmet, who initiated and led the research. His eyes were twinkling, and to my great relief he suddenly uncorked a wave of laughter which rippled all around the table. Maybe the stamp, no doubt banged on the file by some enthusiastic secretary, had engendered in everybody who read it a conviction that he assuredly was not the person to handle such sensitive material. Maybe the system had finally collapsed; designed to soothe bureaucratic breasts rather than to stimulate action, its bluff was finally called. By now it was clear to everyone in the room what I had known for twelve months: no one had answered any of my letters at all.

It was Dr. Faghih, dean of the School of Public Health in Tehran, who finally moved to retrieve the situation, and he did so with that disarming blend of Iranian charm and sweet reasonableness that I was to encounter over and over again and always find endearing. It is an attitude which, while never admitting the existence of a problem, nevertheless does admit the existence of ruffled feelings which must be soothed. "You must please understand, Dr. Goodfield," he said, "that we regarded your visit to us of the greatest importance. You can see for yourself, for we have marked your file *Confidential.* We decided that when you arrived we would be extremely nice to you, and now that you have arrived we are going to be extremely nice to you. What would you like to see?"

Five days later and early in the morning, I left Tehran with Janez Kmet, in a Land Rover supplied by the School of Public Health. We were going up to the Caspian, then to the northeastern provinces to visit the seminomadic tribes who live on the borders of Soviet Central Asia. They are the Turkomans, the people with the highest rate of oesophageal cancer in the whole world.

Oesophageal cancer is one of the nastiest malignancies, extremely painful and slow to develop. If bypass devices are not constructed, the oesophagus gradually becomes more restricted and death comes finally from starvation or thirst. It is not unique to the Turkomans, for it is also very common among

males in Brittany and can be found in both sexes from many
ethnic groups in eastern and southern Africa. It exists in the
Western world too, and though it is one of the minor cancers as
far as numbers are concerned, it is beginning to increase among
the black population of the United States. But there is a very
large belt of this disease which begins in eastern Turkey and
spreads through Iran, then extends eastward into the Soviet
Union and ultimately into Mongolia and northern China.
Amongst the Turkomans in northern Iran and the Kazakhs, who
live on the northeastern shores of the Caspian Sea, it reaches the
highest levels ever recorded. If other causes of death were
prevented, then one in six adults—men and women—would die
of this cancer before the age of sixty-two. Like a sword of
Damocles it hangs over the community of some three hundred
thousand Turkomans in Iran.

Why do these people, in this place, have this terrible level of
the disease, whereas down the road—as it were—other people
from other ethnic groups don't? The answer to this question will
come from epidemiology, a very old science indeed, almost as
old as the cancer itself. The method of this science has been the
most ancient and fundamental in medicine. Whether it was
Ramazini, who in 1703 pointed out that breast cancer was high
in Italian nuns yet low in wet nurses—indeed, in all women who
breast-fed their children—or Sir Percival Pott, who in 1775
described cancer of the scrotum as an occupational hazard of
chimney sweeps, or John Snow, who in 1849 identified a certain
water pump in London as the rogue in a cholera outbreak, the
classic methods have been the same. The idea is to reduce all
variables to one and try to establish this as the cause of the
disease. You ask very specific questions, seeking to reduce and
simplify as you go. You ask a group of smokers: How many
cigarettes a day do you smoke? Do you inhale? For how many
years have you been smoking? Then you compare answers with
those from corresponding groups who never have smoked or who
have given it up.

By their very nature epidemiological studies are quite different from laboratory studies. At the workbench, once a
scientist has a problem and has framed a self-contained question, he can dream up an idea or create a hypothesis. Then he
sets up neat, tightly controlled experiments with mice or fruit

flies, shifting the variables from situation to situation. Eventually he either confirms his idea or he doesn't. Epidemiology isn't like that at all. A scientist has to take the facts, the people, as he finds them, and then sift through the data, searching for correlations, trying to extract the patterns which may suggest relationships between a disease and one or more underlying environmental factors. There are few experiments that can be done. Controls are not totally impossible, but they can be very difficult to arrange. The amalgam of our cultures, the shifting patterns of populations and the complicated overlay of twentieth-century life make it very difficult to isolate communities for enough time to decipher the extrinsic and intrinsic factors at play in the patterns of disease.

That both the right conditions and control groups exist around the Caspian Littoral is a real piece of luck as far as this disease is concerned. Probably nowhere else in the world do such conditions exist. The distance that the research teams must cover is some 1,000 miles. Within this range are groups of people still living in simple, man-soil relationships with the earth, largely dependent upon food grown locally, still quite isolated from the multifarious influences of twentieth-century life. Another important characteristic is that there are striking differences of climate within a few miles, that are reflected in the vegetation, which is in turn mirrored in the pattern of people's lives. One day I was sitting on the floor of a wooden hut in the forests of the Caspian, listening to the rain pelting down outside and talking with the people of water and mud. For centuries now they have cleared small areas in the forest and planted rice, their basic food. Not so many years ago when they were offered bread for the first time they did not recognize it. But only two days before and less than three hundred miles away I had been sitting on a carpet in a tent in the desert, pouring with sweat and talking with the nomads of the loess. When they find water, they stay long enough to grow cereals, and their basic food is bread. The first group has an incidence of oesophageal cancer which is quite ordinary; the second has a rate so high as to be baffling. It is tempting to think—and how convenient it would be—that the difference between little cancer in the first group and much in the second is related to the differences between rain and sun, mud and dust, rice and bread.

But there seems to be no one factor responsible; neither smoking nor carpet-making nor food nor habits. The causes, as yet to be determined, are clearly very complicated and perhaps even very fundamental.

This problem may call for totally new ideas, and the rationale behind the work of Dr. Janez Kmet is quite different from that implicit in the classical approach. He is taking the position of devil's advocate. As he points out, stomach cancer is disappearing from Western life, and to a smaller extent oesophageal cancer too, and doing so during a time of terrible industrial pollution—disappearing in spite of it. Given this, it is perhaps unwise to take an oversimplistic view—to say that just *one* "thing" is *always* the cause of *this* cancer, and the absence of this "thing" will cause it to disappear. Precise chemical causes of cancer, where established, may simply be aberrant features in the history of man, for it is only late in his evolutionary history that he has begun to paint his lungs with tar, ingest asbestos, expose his bladder to aniline dyes and contaminate his food. Perhaps all that the studies of such cancers will tell us is that it is indeed unwise to do these things. But what can such studies tell us about man's fundamental biological condition, those basic factors in life that may make us susceptible to certain diseases?

Janez believes that certain cancers are deeply rooted in our evolutionary past, in the ecology and history of populations as they have developed through time and that the mechanisms of these cancers are equally deeply rooted. He is perfectly aware that he is bucking the well-established trends, though he is not as isolated in his views as he sometimes thinks. With a cancer like cancer of the oesophagus, which is obviously contained within one or more specific groups, it is reasonable to suppose that its repeated expression reflects not only the life history of its victim but also the past history of the population. It is an old cancer in every sense of the word, old in history and old in evolution, possibly a naturally occurring cancer. A Persian physician, Jurjani, described it as far back as the thirteenth century; he too found it amongst the nomadic tribes who inhabited the northeastern provinces, and the mere fact that he mentioned it in those days is itself a measure of the frequency and impact. So cancer of the oesophagus is not just a product of the twentieth-century life; it has been around for very much longer. If, indeed, it reflects a basic relationship between man and his environment, then a detailed study may tell us something very fundamental about ourselves. If we could begin to understand the interplay between our external world and our internal physiological state—both genetically and metabolically—with respect to something like oesophageal cancer, then perhaps we might hope eventually to understand more about the basic conditions that lead to all diseases of this kind.

Janez's effort will be a lengthy one, for epidemiological studies take a lot of time. It may well be a decade before any significant results emerge. As I learned more and more about this most unusual experiment, I was consistently warned about the tentativeness, perhaps even the absence, of results. The researchers ultimately expect to demonstrate the constellation of factors, genetic and environmental, that are at work, but they cannot identify these yet. But I was to see the unique methods by which they were expecting to reveal them.

Listening to Janez's own personal history, I feel it was almost inevitable that he finally ended up in Iran, studying the Turkomans. He is a Yugoslav who until recently has been working at the International Agency for Research on Cancer in Lyons, France. Tall, erect, with white hair and a bushy mustache, he is often mistaken for a British army officer of the nicest type. During the war he was a Partisan and worked with the guerrillas, so it was no surprise to learn from his colleagues that at fifty-seven he spends his free time practically running straight up nine-thousand-foot mountains.

He qualified as a doctor at Zagreb University, and after the war was over he spent a few years in Moscow, working on the control of infectious diseases. He moved naturally into epidemiology, the study of epidemics in their patterns and outcomes; then in 1958 he turned his attention to cancer, which was for him the "last great disease" in man. After ten months at the Sloan-Kettering Institute for Cancer Research in New York, he joined the World Health Organization at Geneva. Finally he took over their oral cancer unit in southeast Asia and spent two years in Soviet Central Asia, India and Ceylon.

It was during his time in Soviet Central Asia that he became intrigued with the problem of oesophageal cancer. The first, precise statistics about the disease in Asia had come from Kazakhstan, so Janez tried to work on the problem there but could not get permission. In 1966 the World Health Organization sent him to Iran to look at the situation there, and while there he read Sir Roger Steven's *The Land of the Great Sophy,* a delightful vignette of the country by a former British ambassador. This book probably marks the beginning of Janez's love affair—for that is what it amounts to—with the region of the Caspian rain belt. He then visited Oxford to talk with Sir Richard Doll, who did the classic scientific studies that implicate smoking as a cause of lung cancer, and it was Doll who emphasized the most interesting, and perhaps the most important, feature about cancer of the oesophagus—the very sharp borderlines between areas of high and low incidence.

So when in November 1966 Janez came from India to Iran on a reconnaissance trip, he was looking for just such cutoff points. He began at Gonbad, a small town on the borders of the Turkoman area, and with the local medical officer went up to the desert, to the lands of the nomadic tribes, where he was later to take me. Then, retracing his steps westward along the Caspian, he looked for the place where there would be a sharp break in the incidence of cancer. He found it at a small town, Nowshahr, right on the edge of the Caspian Sea. Later records made over three years show that in the province of Mazandaran, on the eastern side of the Caspian, six hundred and forty-three cases of this cancer were recorded in men, and five hundred and nineteen in women. By contrast, in Gilan, a province on the western side, records for the same period reveal only one hundred and forty-six cases in men, and forty-six in women. The drop from over one thousand to under two hundred is amazing by any standards.

The next step was to get genuine, watertight statistical information, so with money from the Iranian Public Health Institute and W.H.O., he organized a Cancer Registry throughout the Caspian Littoral. The organization of this registry, a vital prerequisite for the research, was a remarkable feat. Janez needed reliable statistical information, but his sources could not be the carefully ordered, computerized records of hospitals, nor the files of numbers of doctors working with a relatively few patients over a small geographical area. He had to cull information from a wide area in a part of Iran where, at that time, there were only some five hundred doctors, with a ratio of one physician for every eight thousand patients. There were no local pathology services and no large medical centers.

It was clear that even where the hospitals existed, their records would provide very limited information, for oesophageal cancer is so common in the area that it is recognized both as a disease and as invariably fatal. Turkomans might indeed travel great distances to see a physician—perhaps travel again for a second opinion. Occasionally they might be persuaded to go to a town and visit a radiologist. However, once they have a suspicion of oesophageal cancer, they most often prefer to return home to die, instead of expending further engery and expense in extensive investigations or palliative treatment. Thus only the doctor first seen might have knowledge of the case.

So Janez and his Iranian colleagues began at the grass roots. The director of the Public Health Institute in Tehran sent a personal letter to all the doctors in the areas, explaining the project and asking for help. Each doctor was visited by the local medical officer in charge of registry and given cancer notification forms. Every four to six weeks these were collected personally by technicians who checked carefully to make certain that all the doctors, however remote, were visited regularly. In return, the Iranian health authorities established a pathological laboratory at the Babol Research Station. The medical officers met regularly and discussed the problem with the local doctors; lectures were given by visiting specialists in a medical *quid pro quo*, so extending everyone's understanding of the problem. After four years' work, the pattern slowly emerged from the background, and Janez could appreciate the complexity of his problem.

Once the cancer registry was properly established, the team was able to go into the second stage of their work, building up a general picture of the environment. This study covered rainfall, soil analysis, vegetation and agricultural practices—in other words, every kind of environmental detail—until finally the whole area was divided into eight ecological regions with more or less well-defined boundaries. During 1969–70, the first systematic collection of demographic information began, and this was helped immeasurably by a veritable treasure chest of information, the *Iranian Village Gazetteer*. Looking over this *Gazetteer*, I realized how very dull indeed are the census records of England and America, for all the interesting material is missing. The 1966 census in Iran took in every piece of information that it could, covering not only the usual mundane details of ages, births, marriages and deaths, but also two hundred other characteristics, the minutiae of people: the number of shops in a village; the number of teahouses, of tinsmiths, of carpenters; the schools, the *hammams*, the morgues; the variety of occupations; the number of horses, of camels, of donkeys; the location and types of the carpet industry; the crops grown, eaten, and sold; the tools available. From this battery of information, the researchers, particularly Dr. Paula Cook, the team's medical geographer, were able to produce over a hundred maps showing the distribution of a whole range of social and economic features.

The next step was to superimpose all the separate aspects: the incidence of oesophageal cancer, the specific details of the environment, and the social and economic picture. Fusing these, Dr. Cook and Dr. Day, the chief statistician from Lyons, divided the area again into fifteen study-regions. Within these areas of ecological neatness they could identify crucial groups of people, living in islands of simplicity surrounded by the ocean of twentieth-century life that is rapidly engulfing the towns. Then, by looking at a combination of cancer incidence and ecological structure, they were able to focus on three villages in each region as being the best for detailed study.

To get to this point had taken about six years, dating from Janez's first visit to the Caspian in 1966.

This is where I came in. Janez gave me this background on our first morning, during the six-hour drive over the Elburz mountains to Babol. Words are no substitute for sight, and it was only after seeing the Caspian landscape that I came to realize how unique the area is. One is in the mountains immediately after leaving Tehran. Indeed, the city itself, an urban stream of concrete lava, flows down the side of a mountain until it spills dry and desiccated into the plain some two thousand feet below. The Elburz form both a glorious backdrop to the frenetic city and a barrier separating the deserts of the south from the rains and winds of the north. It is this range, hundreds of miles wide with peaks rising to over 12,000 feet, which provides the vital clue to our understanding of the lands and the people. Much of the country in the Elburz is still unexplored, with some of the most glorious and rugged scenery in the world, and like a vigilant sentry the perfect peak of Mount Damevand, soaring to over 17,000 feet, dominates the land.

If one looks at a satellite photograph of the area, from the Soviet Union south into Tehran, this mountainous barrier is covered by a blanket of sickle-shaped cloud permanently laid on the hills. The water vapor surges up from the vast inland sea and forms depressions which break against the mountains, beating against barricades they cannot storm. The clouds precipitate almost immediately and the extent of the rainfall is reflected in the fields and forest below. As we drove in from the south, I became aware of the sharpest ecological change I had ever seen. Within a mile of stark, brown hills, suddenly there were trees, then woods and then forests. Move to the east, toward the desert provinces, and the picture reverses just as quickly. The vegetation changes from tea plantations to rice paddies to open walnut woods to fruit and vegetables to cereals to nothing, and finally the mountains are quite bare again. Between Rasht on the coastal strip, and Moraveh-Tappeh, the northeasternmost point of our journey, near the border of the U.S.S.R., the annual rainfall drops away from some two thousand millimeters a year to two hundred, and all in the space of three hundred and fifty miles.

At Babol, on that first day in a small Persian house, which is the team's headquarters, I met many of the other people concerned with the research: the drivers, pathologists, mechanics, technicians, clerical assistants and Dr. Aramesh, who for this one season was the field coordinator.

When I visited them in 1973, the first real year of detailed study was just finished, yet even this was just preliminary work—just the beginning of Janez's study. In the days that followed I got just a glimpse of this unique bit of scientific research. It is unique in several respects: both because of the problem and its location, and because of the international quality of the supporting agencies, and the work force; Yugoslav, English, American, French, and of course many Iranians.

There are five research teams at work. The first one acts as the reconnaissance team, responsible for contacting local officials in towns, explaining the project to the villages, completing the census and finding a campsite for the other teams. The second two teams, led by Dr. Ing Hormozdiary, collect all possible information on village, household and individual characteristics and the nutritional habits of the people under study. The two clinical teams take the "picture" of the internal environment of the people by a battery of clinical tests. By the time one has added the drivers, cooks, mechanics, technicians and doctors, each team consists of seven to twelve people. They carry their own tents and their own food, and in no way do they depend upon or demand anything from the villagers. At any time during the season they can be found spread out over a distance of 1,000 miles. Dr. Aramesh, who is a very precise and careful man, would, I felt, have loved to have been able to say at any given moment where they all were, people and equipment. But in the absence of walkie-talkies he could never be quite certain. In the Caspian the rains keep coming, so team B2 is bogged down in a foot of mud in one place, and the work schedule is thrown out by a day or so while they dig out the tents or the Land Rover. The supplies have to come up from Tehran: hypodermic needles, sterilized containers to hold the specimens, dry ice to keep them cool. Did those specimens get to Tehran and finally to Canberra? Who *has* the dry ice? Where are the liquid nitrogen containers? The third Land Rover has broken down— how can we get Mr. Moghadan to Tehran and back today? We *must* have a woman interviewer here! We *can't* get up to this village this week! The whole operation forms a crazy kaleidoscope. The transport of people and equipment pose logistic problems worthy of a major expedition into the Himalayas, but whereas in a Himalayan expedition a batch of people is moved from one point to another, and that is the end of the matter, here groups of people have to be back and forth all over the place, hopefully in succession and hopefully in phase. As the extent of the detailed problems impressed itself on my mind, I wondered how they possibly managed. But they manage beautifully, and one gets the feeling of an operation which has swung into its stride, where a sense of perspective and of purpose has prevented people from losing their sense of humor.

The studies in each village are identical. First is a survey of general food and agricultural habits, set against the previous general environmental studies, with everyone in the village being questioned. Then six households ranging across the social stratification that is found even within the smallest communities are selected for a nutritional survey covering food consumption and food intake in the most exact detail. The work of the clinical teams is equally comprehensive: specimens for laboratory analysis are taken from all the villagers, and a clinical examination is given to everyone in the six households. In addition, a second clinical team focuses on both control households and on the households of recently reported oesophageal cancer patients, repeating all the previous tests *in toto*.

The whole procedure is not only complex, it is also highly sensitive, posing problems of a delicate and humane kind. The importation, however temporary, of obtrusive groups of strangers into a stable pattern of life can be catastrophic if not handled with insight and delicacy. Even a disruption of tempo can be unsettling. Being an object of scrutiny can be unnerving even for the most carefree of us, and worse, this can precipitate a deluge of fears and anxieties if we don't know what is going on. Everything possible is done to minimize disruptions and draw the people into an understanding of the work. Authoritarian attitudes on the part of the civil health authorities, or patronizing ones on the part of the scientists, would be not only obnoxious, but self-defeating. In any case, Janez wouldn't stand for it. Every day that I observed him observing them, and watched his minute-to-minute handling of problems, I felt that he considered it his undeserved fortune to work with these people, rather than their privilege to have their affliction an object of scientific study. His scruples are no doubt bolstered by the painful realization that he is doing nothing for them. The work may perhaps benefit the next generation of Turkomans, but the present one must continue to live with the hovering presence of this cancer, just as their ancestors did in the past. One consequence of his humane sensitivity, however, is that everybody seems to adore him, research teams and Turkomans alike. As we visited the villages and the W.H.O. Land Rover screeched to a halt in a settlement, we would be either engulfed by a crowd of excited children or welcomed with quiet dignity by a few adults. Time and time again I saw the faces light up when it was realized that Janez had come. The man and his work are clearly accepted now as a part of the pattern of life, and this alone is an enormous achievement.

Though I managed to see every team and each type of village under study, I missed what is obviously the best, the essential touch of theater, when the reconnaisance team, in the first phase, attempts to "move in" on a village. The scene was described to me, however. The formalities begin, the rituals which must be gone through at the local government level before the research teams can come. They pay their respects to the local governor of the district, and armed with a letter from him, they then call on the local head of the gendarmes. Armed now with another letter, they pay a formal visit to the head of the village, the *Kadkhoda*. His title literally means "the hand of God," and though I don't know how he is chosen, it conjures up visions of apostolic succession. The *Kadkhoda* calls a village meeting, held in the mosque or the school, which is attended by the men of the village and the doctors from the local town. The main inspirational address, for this is what it amounts to, is given by one of the senior technicians, Mr. Deirmina, an old hand of the institute, who adores public speaking. With qualities of warmth and eloquence, he both captivates and convinces. He reminds the villagers of something they know perfectly well, that there are many people among them with a disease that catches them in the throat. The problem is, first, to find out why this disease appears, as a preliminary to finding a cure. So people will be coming from the medical schools to do some investigations, with the help of the local doctors they already know. He emphasizes, several times, that the investigations have nothing to do with malaria, security or tax. While the precise order in which these assurances are given is irrelevant, the assurances themselves are very necessary, I was told, for malaria, security and tax form a most unholy trinity of afflictions which has plagued the people of the Caspian Littoral for generations. At least the malaria is now completely controlled: after the war the Iranian government launched a classically successful malarial eradication program. As a result Janez's team inherited both a vast capital of good will and a medical structure which greatly eased their own problems of organizing this enormous field study.

Before we went up to the Turkoman area I saw the work of the nutritional teams in the intermediate areas between forest and desert, at two control villages a few miles from Babol with populations of 136 and 223 people. The settlements straggled out along a track of deep, wet mud, with fast-flowing streams on either side. The landscape was rich and heavily wooded, with lush water meadows and fields of rice. The team's camp, a large one, was set some way back from the village in a wetly luxuriant field where the essence of thyme and mint was ground out underfoot. Each team was completely self-contained and self-supporting, striking a delicate balance: trying to establish the best possible contact with the villagers without depending on them in any way. Village life went on as normally as possible, with a quiet overlay of research activity; people were questioned around their usual activities or in their houses. Initially the teams tried to keep to the agricultural calendar and avoid visiting the villages during the period of most active work in the fields. In practice, however, this would have meant leaving out the spring and summer season—all very well, but in the winter too many of the villages are inaccessible through the mud. So now in spring and summer research is concentrated mostly into the early morning or evening hours. This was how we found the team, working in the twilight. I remember the eerie feeling as we walked in single file across the rice paddies, into a moist darkness and enveloping quietness. It was, as Janez joked, good guerrilla country.

These first teams make two basic surveys, directed by a couple of nutritionists and a female assistant, while two trained interviewers and translators complete the village and household questionnaires. It is like a vast fact-finding market survey. Janez and Paula Cook have worked out a whole battery of questions in English that have been translated into Farsi, with the other minority languages and dialects being covered by listing certain key words, for there is still a fair ethnic mixing among these communities. The questions cover as many facets as possible: how many people are there in the household, what are their ages, when do they get up in the morning, what do they do throughout the hours of the day; do they clean their teeth, and how; what do they eat and when; are there certain foods they avoid or take specially, and why; how do they store their milk products; what clothes or rugs do they make at home, what dyes are used; do they take or make any homemade medicines; what is in them; what are their common ailments; do they use any alcohol, opium or tobacco.

I stood in on the procedure of one questionnaire—stood, not sat, for the interview took place in the middle of the main mud track. A student from the Nutritional Institute in Tehran was talking with a young woman, caught briefly between chores, and though they were both the same age she was addressing the interviewee as "Mother." The woman was barefooted in the mud, with a sleeping baby across her back. Her skin was stained brown from walnuts, her teeth were riddled with gold fillings and her clothes were startlingly bright. The effect was of an exotic bird in a tropical rain forest. There was an obvious rapport between interviewer and interviewed: they were laughing a great deal together. Perhaps the deceptive silliness of some of the questions struck them both. As he listened to them, Janez began to laugh too and explained that they were in amongst the usual hazards of ambiguity in questionnaires, scientific or advertising. For example, the question "Do you drink your tea hot, warm or cold?" was always countered with a scornful "Who would drink cold tea?" a most reasonable answer. Consequently the teams are now having to do a special study of tea temperature, with built-in thermometers in cups. Other questions are not only apparently stupid but could possibly be quite provocative. There is enough tobacco and opium and alcohol around to make questions about them reasonable, but it quickly became apparent that questions about alcohol directed to women were unreasonable, provoking the same kind of outraged shock that would be forthcoming if one asked the most reactionary of matrons in any country how many times a week she smoked grass. Certain issues must be approached by something less than the direct method.

The detailed nutritional studies in the households are conducted with the same care that is brought to bear on the diet of a diabetic. For five days one girl will remain with each of the selected households, watching not only what they eat but also the way they cook, weighing out the food with the wife and covering all details of her procedure. I was taken to see one of these households in the average range of the social hierarchy, a farmer with a small amount of personal land. The small houses stretched out on either side of the track are set back on the other side of the stream and hidden behind an equally small mud wall. I felt a curious Gulliver-in-Lilliput sensation as I went in. A small step got me over the moat and the stream, then with another I entered the gatehouse through a small wooden door in the mud wall. Having penetrated these toylike fortifications, I was in a courtyard with the two-storied wooden house facing me. We climbed up the outside stair onto the balcony and were invited into the main, and only, room. Rust mats covered the floor; the walls were mud and wattle—painted over with a bright blue wash. We removed our shoes and joined the two women sitting cross-legged on the floor. Between them there was a pair of scales, a basket of rice, some eggs and a pan. "How much rice for this evening?" she asked. Four portions were scooped out and the nutritionist weighed it. "Anything else?" An egg was added to the pile, then the water was measured. A few green leaves from the meadow—spinachlike—were added, and these, with tea, made up supper for the household of four. Backing these food studies, water samples from the stream and soil samples from the earth are also scanned and analyzed. The chemical background of these peoples' lives, in all its fine detail, is ultimately recorded and stored on computer with every quantum of information on hand.

The Turkomans, the real focus of this study, were two days away from Babol in a remote, but fascinating, region where space is still measured by time rather than by distance. The people must walk for five or six days to take their sheep and carpets, their main source of capital, to market. It took us two days of hard driving to get to them and a third exhausting day of battering before we reached the groups with the highest incidence of cancer. That final day we covered one hundred kilometers in fourteen hours, lurching slowly through the desert toward the borders of the Soviet Union, driving along uneven, bumpy tracks of packed sand with deep corrugations that could easily flip a Land Rover onto its side. We headed north, then

northeast, and it became progressively hotter and drier and
dustier as we climbed up to the plateau.

The Turkoman's desert is like no other landscape I have seen.
It is not the stylized mixture of flat sand alternating with long
undulating dunes that is so familiar to us, nor is it "range upon
range of hills," a misleading description since the heights are not
mountains nor even hills. Most accurately one should use the
word "loess," a technical term for a feature formed by blown
sands compacting hard and firm over thousands of years. Here
these had been blown, then fiercely driven, by the winds from
the northern steppes, icy in winter, parching in summer. What is
finally formed is something less than hills, but larger than
hillocks, and once in among these geological pimples you can
see neither around nor over them. It is impossible to fix on a
landmark, and at one stage we were quite lost, so Janez, our
driver and our interpreter kept watchful eyes on the mountains
of the Soviet Union to orientate us. Though Janez and I made
plenty of jokes about stumbling into Russia, our companions
were both visibly nervous; I think they found such jokes in
slightly bad taste. Our horizon was only some forty miles
through the heat haze, but this particular stretch of loess goes on
for some five hundred miles into the Soviet Union, ending in the
biggest desert in all central Asia. Beyond that, again, is another
area of loess, and beyond that, more desert, then finally China.
Dry and stark, it is a harsh environment. Apart from a few birds
of prey, camels were the only animals we saw—singly, then in
groups, and finally in an enormous herd of some two hundred,
which we smelled long before we saw them. They were searching
as the nomads search, for telltale flashes of green, where a small
amount of water might support a small amount of grass.

One never quite knows where the tribes themselves will be
found. Though there are semipermanent settlements, the Turkomans still preserve something of their nomadic pattern of life.
In the warm months they pick up their tents and herds and
wander, looking for grazing and water. Then they plant wheat
and stay till it can be harvested. So we stumbled upon my first
Turkomans, spotting the characteristic circular tents from some
distance away. We left the track and drove across the sand to be
met by a group of nervous children, who had never seen the

W.H.O. vehicle before, and four furry dogs. Janez and the interpreter slowly got down and greeted them, but I didn't move. I had earlier been made to promise not to leave the Land Rover until all the dogs were tethered. They are large and vicious.

Gradually people gathered around, and we moved to where a tent was being raised—the carpet already on the floor, the felt walls and roof braided and tied to the circular skeleton of poles. The tents are their symbol of an ancient mobility. These tribes were once completely fluid, flowing like streams all over central Asia. Thus it is not surprising that this same cancer afflicts the Turkomans in the central areas of the Soviet Union also, and in China as well. According to legend, Alexander the Great had come this way and had built a large mud wall running west to east to keep out the barbarians—which in effect meant the Turkomans. Even as recently as fifty years ago they would sweep down from the steppes and raze the Persian villages; raping, pillaging—all the time-honored verbs applied. They could dismantle their tents so rapidly that whole villages could disappear within an hour and the tribes be lost and gone away. But now national attitudes have solidified natural boundaries; across the border in the Soviet Union, the Turkomans have been settled into the towns. But when Janez looks north he does so with a real regret, one compounded, I think, of clinical interest and natural wanderlust.

As the crowd gathered—the women in superbly colored robes and *chador*, the men with their rectangular lamb hats—I could easily see the Chinese features in their faces, made even more marked by the thin, wispy Mongolian beards. The ancient mobility was reflected in their faces too. It would have been possible to have lined twenty people in a row and cover the whole spectrum of ethnic groups from western Turkey to the China Seas. The men were tall, quiet and immensely dignified, the women cheerful but remote, routinely working in a manner long tried, never questioned. I sensed something both persistent and sad about them all. Persistent because the history of these people was still tangible, a proud background proclaimed by their present proud bearing. Yet it is a history which carries a terrible disease which any one of them there could be starting to show. Sad, too, because without wishing to romanticize the primitive ways of life, one could sense that they were aware of the dilution of their history, of a gradual weakening of autonomy and a loss of identity, as compared to the days when they could wander freely over thousands of square miles. The Turkomans may finally disappear, assimilated into the wider culture. I hope not. Before they do, however, they may perhaps have something to tell us all about community or about dying in quiet relationship with the universe, and if Janez is right, there is something very specific that they can tell us about disease, too.

As I looked at the landscape again and then at the people whose pattern of life and deep structure Janez was trying to capture, my feelings began to move in a cycle which I was to experience several times more in the next nine months: alternating spirals of impotence and hope. I remembered the correspondence in *Science*, provoked by an article written by Janez and his Iranian colleague, Ezattollah Mahboubi. Someone pressed on the issue of psychosomatic influences as a factor in cancer, suggesting that the question Janez really should be asking was "For how many months before you first felt the symptoms were you feeling unhappy or depressed?" It is of course a thoroughly leading question, designed to promote the answer you want rather than the real one, but I looked at these people knowing that such a question might well make no sense to them at all. Perhaps they *were* unhappy, but how could they express this? In any case, there is such an acceptance, born out of the recognized inevitability of their pattern of life, that the question is made meaningless. The routine of chores is all: work matched to the cycles of the seasons, crops to be grown, tents and animals to be moved, bread to be baked, carpets to be woven, children to be born, life to be survived, disease to be endured, and death to be met.

As I watched the interaction between the Yugoslav scientist and the Turkomans, I found the moment very powerful, for both the Turkomans' past and Janez's problem have a similar profundity. The core of science is the same everywhere, whether in a laboratory or in a desert. Nature is dumb. A scientist goes to the world and asks those questions that, on the basis of both intuitive feelings and experience, he hopes are the right ones. But if the world itself is silent so, too, are the Turkomans. They cannot speak for themselves for they have no tradition of medical knowledge; they can only tell us about their human experience of pain. How could Janez possibly know where to look: how could he be sure that he was asking the right questions? He cannot ever tell in advance. When all the data has accumulated, and if on examination patterns emerge which point to the internal and external causes of this cancer, only then will Janez know if his method has worked.

If they are isolated, so too was he. This remarkable work and its execution stemmed basically from this one man, and it has imposed on him a degree of isolation which he confesses has become almost unbearable at times, strong though he is. There has been the usual loneliness of any pioneer exploring a new intellectual frontier in the face of incredulity or skepticism, but this project has demanded a physical and mental loneliness of another sort as well. For eight years before the groups became assembled, Janez spent much of his time here, miles from anywhere, in an alien culture with no one to whom he could talk or with whom he could argue or just unwind. People are willing to make many sacrifices for their science; his were quite different from those of any of the other cancer scientists I met.

I now saw the second arm of the research: the gathering of extensive clinical data in the Turkoman villages. There are a few settlements immediately to the east of the Caspian Sea, on the vast alluvial plain—the original sea bottom—which now separates the water from the desert. At six o'clock one morning we drove into a small village strung out near the Gorgan River, which empties in the Caspian. Outside the village a thin young man flagged us down. He had that tall, dark, handsome look of so many Persians, and was a draftee doing his military service by working in the rural areas on projects such as this. This is one of the eminently sensible alternatives to the draft that is available in Iran: a man can go to the country and teach in the literary programs, or he can do paramedical work amongst the tribes, or he can join the afforestation teams. He was bubbling with delight to see Janez, and ran ahead to tell the teams we were coming. The whole population seemed to be up and around, and crowds of excited children flowed around the Land Rover, which, like a mechanical Pied Piper, slowly led us all to the schoolhouse.

The camp was set up nearby: tents for sleeping, relaxing, cooking, eating, supplies, clinics, laboratory, and toilets. Generators, heaters and fans were lined up with vehicles, those ubiquitous Land Rovers whose engines would both transport the teams and generate light and power for the laboratory equipment. The clinical team, two doctors, a female technician for the electrocardiograph and three laboratory technicians were in the schoolhouse. They had all risen as early as we had, four o'clock, and at five had begun work in a fifteen-hour workday that would stretch until eight that night. Janez slipped into the school, then returned and told me to come inside, where a young Turkoman was having an electrocardiogram examination. He would, he said, introduce me to the girl, her mother, and the leader of the team, Dr. Shahbasi, and ask if I might talk with them. "But judge for yourself the right moment to leave," he warned.

We spoke to them first from behind the curtain, then went in; Janez introduced me, then left. As we entered, the girl on the couch, just about to be fitted to the leads, immediately seized her *chador*, the tentlike veil, and placed one corner in her mouth, where it would remain all the time I was there. None of the women in Iran are fully veiled now, so the face is never completely covered, but amongst the nomads this symbolic act of biting the veil in the presence of strangers is a cultural diminutive from the earlier days. As the ECG machine droned, she smiled at me once or twice. She was twenty-four, married, but had no children. Her mother, sitting rigid and formal, was very much in charge of everything: she neither bit the veil nor smiled, but her eyes constantly flitted between me and her daughter and the doctor and the technician. I sensed that it would be politic to stay only a few minutes—I asked one or two questions. They asked me some, too: where did I come from; why had I travelled so far from my home; what was I doing in their desert; why was I asking all these questions? Then I left. The doctor said he would be out presently.

While we were waiting Janez introduced me to the *Kadkhoda* and some of the other village elders. They explained that they were always happy to see the teams and to work with them. In these situations it is difficult to know whether it is politeness and politics that dictate such words, but in this case I don't think so, as the working partnership seemed to me to be a very genuine one. Several months later and in another desert eight hundred miles to the south, I heard the same feelings expressed most poignantly by the Baktiari, who were delighted with the new paramedical programs there. For centuries now, these nomads have had to take their chances, medically speaking, and they have known only too well what this implies. The cold statistic— one in six men and women dead—when applied to the living group of forty-eight or so around us, meant that I could flick my eye over them like a cold, malevolent deity and decide arbitrarily which eight would simply be snuffed out. But worse: they wouldn't just be snuffed out. Over twenty years the symptoms would slowly develop and intensify till there was only opium to relieve the pain and nothing to relieve the thirst or hunger or the dread certainty that you were the current victim of the tribal scourge. Even the fact that someone recognized the problem and was beginning to do something must by itself have seemed miraculous after centuries of ignorance and indifference. Politeness or politics, there would be no reason to be anything but sincere in this situation.

Though it was only seven o'clock in the morning, the temperature in the shade was already 95° F. By noon it would be 113° F. and 122° F. in the tents. The doctors came out into the shade of the schoolhouse to rest for a while and tell me what was going on. The clinical tests are as penetrating as the nutritional ones. During the course of a physical examination the doctors first look for signs of deficiencies, whether of protein, calories in general or vitamins. They ask questions about any difficulties in swallowing, going back as far as possible into the patient's life history. Blood pressures, measured both by hand and by automatic recorders, are matched into measurements of the heart activity as recorded on the electrocardiograph. Specimens are then taken of saliva, hair and nails, in the search for trace elements—those chemicals which even in the minutest amounts are vital for certain bodily functions. People are given containers and asked to return the next morning with samples of urine and faeces. They are also asked to take no food that morning until blood samples have been drawn.

This ends the villagers' involvement; now the technicians get to work. Many tests can be done immediately in the field, and some of them must be done at once. The urine is tested for sugar, protein and blood, then further prepared for measurements of vital enzymes or traces of opium. The faeces are immediately prepared for examination for intestinal parasites. The haemoglobin content of the blood is measured immediately, and then batches of whole blood, washed red cells, blood serum, plasma and blood clots are separated and stored in containers varying from lunchboxes to liquid nitrogen vials, to ship out to the laboratories. Though these examinations initially cover only the selected households, they take an enormous amount of time. It takes an hour to perform the clinical test for one person and a second hour to go through the laboratory field tests. This was not too bad when only fifteen to twenty people were involved, but now the numbers are increasing fast as more of the population is being covered.

The specimens are then shipped all over the world. The first hair and nail samples go to Glasgow, Scotland, for analysis; some of the blood goes to Canberra, Australia, where immunological and at least thirteen other sophisticated tests can be done. Biochemical knowledge of blood fluid is now so precise that the state of various elements in the blood can be seen to mirror the biological activity of the various organs. If it is important to know about the activity of the bone marrow, a test for iron in the blood serum will reveal this. If it is suspected that the liver is damaged, then a serum gammaglutamyl transpeptidase (S.G.T.P.) test will look for a critical liver enzyme, and so on. It seems neat, exact and straightforward, but science in the desert is never straightforward.

Many things make life difficult for Janez and his teams. Religious customs can hamper, even modify, scientific results unless great care is taken. By Moslem religious custom, nails are kept very short, so samples are difficult to obtain. The women use two different dyes, one red, one black, as hair color; the dyes distort the subsequent chemical analysis. The obvious alternative, the pubic hair, is not so obvious an alternative to the women. In any case, it too is cut right down, so, as custom dictates, "It cannot be tugged out by hand." Then of course the timetables go wrong. The team may arrive and find that their subjects have vanished: only the day before, a large part of the male population may have moved to the summer pastures. The heavy work in the fields may have finished only the evening before, but off they will go to the next job, and the teams must chase after them. By the time they have been run to earth or have returned to the village, another follow-up team may have arrived. Before the routine of a ten-day work cycle, with break days in between, had been established, a delay in one team's work would precipitate a crisis for the next. It was just not possible to have two groups of ten people try to examine one hundred villagers and still let them get on with their daily work.

Then there is the snow or the rain or the mud or the desert. Roads become inaccessible; vehicles break down or get stuck; specimens leak out or spoil because the dry ice has melted; other specimens will freeze and be ruined because too many plastic ice packs were put into a picnic box, and the ice was working only too well. The nutritional teams have their individual purgatories, too. The reasons why all the initial questionnaires were not completed are very revealing. "Shy, would not speak in front of father-in-law," reads the comment on one male from Hottan. Since the father-in-law probably refused to leave, stalemate was inevitable. The categories of "dumb," "senile," "sick in hospital," "mad" or "in prison" tell their own sad story. Others are happier: "left to get married," "away at college," "away on a journey," "too young." All these make gaps that have to be filled in subsequent studies. The kaleidoscope of activity is colorful, but at times it is also confusing and frustrating.

In the days we spent with the Turkomans, I covered all of the scientists' daily activities and those of the tribespeople as well. I saw the men as herders and farmers: the women as makers of carpets and as bakers of bread. The diet is thin and poor; bread is the staple of their diet, with a lot of tea and sometimes a little milk. The women bake four times a day. The ovens are hollowed out of the earth like inverted beehives, and a fire is built at the base. The dough is then slapped onto the walls, and there it remains until the bread is baked. It has no buoyancy at all, and tastes very heavy and stodgy. "Is this really all they eat?" I asked Janez. "Yes," he replied. "There is nothing except bread four times a day. A little tea, possibly meat once a year at a wedding or a feast. You must learn a new scientific concept," he went on, teasingly. "It's 'cellular boredom.' I first heard it from an English scientist who came out last year. So monotonous is their life, so drab is the diet that the cells of the oesophagus just give up the struggle . . . It's simply not worth it!"

I teased him in return. It was a good theory but surely too simplistic for his taste. Turning serious, I began to articulate the questions that I would ask everyone during the next nine months. What combination of factors could we conceive to be at work here? What starts the cancer off? Why does it take so long to develop? Janez didn't really know—no one really knows—but several months later back in Michigan and New York I would begin to perceive a dim outline of a possible answer. Janez's results, gleaned from his treasure chest of data, will take the form of suggestive patterns only; the theory will have to be added later.

One morning, at the wonderfully late hour of seven o'clock, we left the border settlement of Moraveh-Tappeh, and after four days we could at last turn south again, following the ancient tracks of the rapacious Turkoman tribes over the upland plain. There was a hot wind blowing from Russia, and as we drove away from the border I looked back at the mountains of the U.S.S.R., desolate and stark, gashed open by erosion, the chemicals and minerals bursting from the earth. We were driving out of the aridity towards the moisture, and from a long way off we could see the first traces of the rain belt. Two hours out from Moraveh-Tappeh, from the top of the ridge and far away to the south, I saw trees again. Here we dropped our guide and for some unspoken reason waited and watched until he shrank into the landscape. I watched him intently, a small figure loping across the hillside, till he vanished behind some rocks. He was walking into a new world, into a new way of life, for he had decided to leave the tribe to join the army. In a real sense, he was also walking away from the cancer, though he could not know this, but his children and his grandchildren might now well not develop it. Then the driver let in the clutch, and the Land Rover moved slowly down the ridge. As we went down, the green of the Caspian came up toward us, spreading over the hillside from the valley below. So we too drove into another world.

The trip ended on a note of pure farce, as I became caught up in what seemed like a Marx Brothers' film, with simultaneous sound track in five languages. It took two days to catch up with the fourth clinical team, the most colorful and polyglot of them all. Last seen and—since they were very voluble—no doubt last heard too, they were heading toward the Caspian shoreline. We drove after them, and as we travelled east, the clouds piled up, the humidity soared, and finally the rains teemed down in torrential cloudbursts. We travelled east from Babol into the area of the tea plantations, Burma by the sea. Here the coastal strip is very narrow and dark-green plantations spill all down the slopes. After many phone calls, discussions and "guesstimates," during which figures concerning likely rainfall were bandied about with E.T.A.'s, we learned that Team Four was somewhere along the shores of the sea. "This is not very precise," Dr. Aramesh said sadly. He had joined us for my last day. The team had been held up by the rains and the mud and couldn't make the schedule up to their village that day, so they were waiting by the sea. They were, Janez warned me, the most "individual" team of all—a "very individual" team—and it was clear that they were his delight. Just beyond Bandar-e Pahlavi, the old port of Enzeli, where nineteenth-century travellers to Persia entered from Russia, we turned onto the shore itself, asking anyone who seemed helpful whether they had seen the W.H.O. Land Rover. We spun along the sand, dodging boats, missing fishermen, avoiding ditches and playing dodgems with the taxis. These were all over the place, for Iranians seem to exercise their machines on the sand as other people do their horses. We peered myopically through the rain as the Land Rover sought its twin, and were alternately euphoric and disheartened. Everything looked horribly uniform.

They had seen us, however—heaven knows how—for as we drove back over the sand after a few miles, we were flagged down by a young technician, his hair streaming with water. Somehow by the usual bush telegraph the word had got through that we were looking for them, so he had left the beach hut and walked through the rain to find us. Their Land Rover was parked way behind the hut and the clinical tent was pitched to one side. Inside, the group was at work, marking up the specimens from two days before and packing the samples into liquid nitrogen, getting them ready for shipment. This team, the essential "case-control" team, works the same exhausting hours as their colleagues in the other clinical group. They concentrate on families with recently reported cancer cases: looking for genetic links, taking the same specimens and doing the same clinical tests both on these people and on an equal number of control families with no known oesophageal cancer. The samples of blood which would go to Canberra might well be the most revealing of all. For the immunological properties of the blood will reveal patterns in genetic background. Finally, in the private quiet of a scientist's mind and in public meetings at Lyons and Tehran, the work of all five groups would be examined and dovetailed together to find that factor, or constellation of factors, which is at work here. There are no solid conclusions yet, but it is likely that all oesophageal cancer victims will be found to have the same genetic make-up. If so, such families could then be screened much earlier and dietary changes prescribed. We know already that this cancer vanishes within two generations when Turkomans become urbanized, though we are not sure why this happens. We could solve their problem by urbanizing them all, but of course this is hardly a humane solution.

We moved into the beach hut. The team had their families with them, and trying to save on their living allowance, they had rented two huts on the shore—for all. The leader of the team, Dr. Nickbin, was a charming young Iranian who had been trained in France, but at the end of the season he was going to Copenhagen for a year's study. Another technician had known Janez for a long time from some earlier studies. He had trained in Germany, and like many other people working on these projects, had got so fascinated by the problem that he hoped to move from the laboratory and eventually become a doctor. Many of the technicians I would meet in future months would go the same way, either to the clinical side or into research. Janez turned to me in mock despair. "Now at last you will see my problem. I must talk Russian, English, French, American, Farsi, German and my own two Yugoslav languages. Wherever they go to train, wherever they are, I must speak their language." We talked for an hour in a polyglot mixture of pidgin Farsi, French, German and English. Under such circumstances international words like "immuno-suppression" and "histo-incompatibility" are like straws to a drowning man, and I clutched at them. Wives and children too crowded into the hut, squatting on the rugs and listening. The surrealism of the languages finally gave way to a teasing, relaxed whimsicality in which science was mingled with four different cultures. But we were all very tired, for it was the end of the research season.

Two more days and my circuit was complete. Back in Tehran I spoke with Janez at length, studied the literature, looked over the maps, examined the photographs and tried to make some sense of it. One evening I went to the British Council to meet Audrey for dinner. Over a drink I started to tell her about the trip. She listened intently and finally began to laugh, for well into my stride, I began expounding "Goodfield's theory" with all the fanaticism of a missionary. I was remembering the country and the driving, and was coming up with the "dust theory of oesophageal cancer"—untried, unproven but perhaps not totally unlikely.

I was stopped in midtrack, however, the theory exploded as all such theories finally are. Unlike many scientists who use daggers to explode those balloons they suspect are filled with hot air, Audrey punctured mine gently. "Well, then, do their horses get it?" she asked flatly. It was a telling objection. I never found any firm information about the Turkoman horses and cancer, but I later learned that in one valley in Kenya where there is a high rate of oesophageal cancer among the tribes, the cows get it. Moreover, they begin to show it at the same stage in their lives as humans; namely, halfway through the life span. It is all very puzzling.

The eight-hour flight from Tehran to London gave me plenty of time for reflection. As the plane banked sharply away on its flight path to the west, I caught a last glimpse of the Elburz range and wondered where the teams were. Were they stuck in mud again, or—the work finally done for the season—had they pulled back to Tehran for the winter? How would it all go in the future? What would the results show? I remembered that Janez had once said to me: "You can speak about what you want to do and you can die of speaking, but no one will care. But if you eventually prove your point, then perhaps they will listen." He was referring to his own research within epidemiology. Without bitterness, but with realistic humor, he admits that the official school doesn't think very much of his overall approach. However, the connections between genetic make-up and susceptibility to certain cancers now being made in places like the Sloan-Kettering Institute will please him, for they are proving one of his points. Both genetics *and* environment are at work here and are probably at work in all cancers. Environmental insults can take advantage of a genetic predisposition, and a cancer is manifested. This is his own line of reasoning, and it is already clear that this rationale may well prove to be true for all cancers. Meanwhile he is trying to open a new door, to follow a new line and see where it will lead. Within the framework of classical epidemiology, he is extending the methods, not supplanting them, moving down the spectrum of sheer empiricism somewhere toward the understanding. Richard Doll has often emphasized that population studies do not tell us how and why a cancer is produced biologically, only that it *is* produced. Classical epidemiology reveals only some of the links in the chains of cause and effect, but Janez expects and hopes that his study will also reveal something about basic biological predispositions.

Whatever the future brings, he has already proved several points, one of which delights me. The trip was an object lesson in research, and also in the necessity of applying critical standards of science to one's own attitudes. Many of us brought up in the Western tradition have adopted a particular rationale for research far too easily. We think that there *must* be a high-powered lab, with costly equipment and everything at hand—whether technicians, patients or specimens—before significant work can be done. The conclusions drawn out of simple situations, however, may be just as valid as those drawn from complicated ones. This adorable, polyglot international team, functioning miles away from the conveniences and accoutrements which are now taken for granted in scientific research, is doing work which is very fundamental. From the point of view of difficulty, the problems of cancer may well be intractable, but they are not insoluble. To solve them, however, options have to be kept open and prejudices held at bay.

Audrey had given me lunch before my flight, and over drinks

one of her colleagues had murmured, "You don't look very well." I didn't feel particularly good; I thought it was a mixture of excitement, travel and work. But by the time we landed at London Airport, the symptoms were unequivocal. Most appropriately, as it turned out, I had caught the local virus.

2

CANCER AND VIRUSES:

THE NASTIEST PROBLEM IN BIOLOGY

THE SYMPTOMS VARY very little: aches, fever, sore throat, congestion, and that "general feeling of discomfort" which is the medical euphemism for feeling awful. The remedy is equally unchanging: bed rest, aspirin and plenty of fluids. You have probably caught a virus. It was Salvador Luria, director of cancer research at Massachusetts Institute of Technology, who characterized the problem of viruses in cancer as the nastiest in biology, and there is a whole spectrum to that nastiness. They can be nasty in their effects, nasty to manipulate, nasty because of their elusiveness, nasty because of their lethalness. But irritating and irretrievable though they may be, the intellectual challenge they present is clearly irresistible. After I had made their acquaintance on the research level—as distinct from a lifelong clinical familiarity—I was tempted once again to parody Henry James talking to Peyton Rous: "To be young and have divine power"; "To be small and be so vicious." A virus can be very vicious: it can carry you off by a massive infection or, as we now suspect, it can do so by cancer.

It is fitting to remember Peyton Rous, for it was his work in 1911 that implicated viruses with cancer. He extracted a fluid from the tumor of a chick and filtered it, an accepted technique for removing large infectious germs. Then he injected this fluid into other birds, starting with the relatives of the original animal. They also developed tumors. He repeated this technique but extended the injections to other hens not related to the first one, then finally to chicks of any breed. As time went on, the tumors he induced got nastier and more malignant, so the next question was obvious: Are cancers caused by viruses? The argument has been going on ever since. Fifty-five years after his experiment, at the age of eighty-seven, Rous was belatedly given the Nobel Prize, and by then the hunt was well and truly underway. The chase still continues, but even after sixty years of research it has not yet been *proven* that viruses are a cause of cancer in *man.* No one has yet managed to isolate or identify such a virus, but they are by now thoroughly implicated, in the same way that a thief is implicated in the robbery of a bank when, large bag of swag in hand, he is surprised by security guards and runs off.

As particle physicists are now chasing the quark, so cancer virologists, intoxicated by grants and enthusiasm, are chasing human cancer viruses. And many, varied and conflicting have been their claims. One gets the sense of the hunt going off in a variety of directions; as the fox briefly shows himself, there is a cry of "Tallyho!" and everyone gallops away. Then the fox appears briefly somewhere else, laying false scents as he moves, and with yet another cry of "Tallyho!" the direction changes again. No one is quite certain, however, whether it is the same fox they are chasing. So inevitably at the end of the day faint cries of "Gone away" come drifting down the evening air. For some time now, the atmosphere in cancer virus research has been an explosive mixture of optimism, energy, wishful thinking, fury and flamboyance. The money has been there, the incentive has been there, but too often the viruses have not. They have been infuriating, and, if anything, the trail has become more baffling the longer the chase has continued.

An enormous amount of money and effort has gone into a

search for a viral cause of cancer. The sense of urgency has been intensified by the startling realization that the SV 40 virus can induce tumors in certain animals. In the 1950's this virus was a contaminant in the cultures of monkey kidney tissues, which were used as a medium to grow the polio virus. At the time there was no reason at all to suspect the cancer-inducing properties of the virus, but the fact remains that a large number of people received an injection of SV 40 along with their polio shot. We know now that viruses behave very differently as they move across animal species, so the risk is very slight, but SV 40 is no longer a permitted contaminant.

Another goad comes from the promise of a vaccine for cancer. Vaccines have been one of the great successes of medical science; thus the possibility of a vaccine is highly tantalizing and intriguing. If it turns out that cancer viruses behave in typical patterns of infection, then in theory the possibility of a cancer vaccine becomes a very real one. If polio and smallpox, why not cancer too? However, once again cancer makes its own rules, for we have not yet managed to identify any virus causing a human cancer with real certainty, nor is there any immediate prospect of a vaccine. This is not because scientists have been slothful or inefficient; it is merely that, as so often happens in science, they have realized that the problem is infinitely more difficult than they at first supposed. During all these years scientists have certainly learned a great deal about viruses and their mode of action, but as Thomas Maugh wrote in a recent article in *Science*, "They have also learnt a great deal about humiliation and credibility."

I looked at one part of this work through the activities of a few people who were concentrating their efforts on one rare cancer, Hodgkin's disease. I did so at the largest and one of the most prestigious cancer research centers in the world, the Sloan-Kettering Institute of New York. Together with Memorial Hospital, this vast, sprawling organization with two research arms—one in Manhattan, another upstate in Rye—is one of the Meccas of cancer. It is a place you have to get to if you are a cancer scientist or a cancer patient, and in either case the competition for a laboratory bench or a hospital bed is fierce. Millions of dollars have flowed in for research, from private and public sources, to irrigate cell biology, immunology, virology—

all those fields in fact that could possibly relate to the one fundamental problem. With such finance and preeminence it can—and does—attract some of the finest research scientists from all over the world. These scientists, with their supporting substructure of doctors, technicians, librarians, security guards, drivers, students and secretaries, form a seething amalgam of idiosyncratic human beings, united not by any abstract law of science or human behavior but rather by the knowledge that their mutual raison d'être is to understand and cure cancer.

For five weeks I was with this one group in the laboratories of Dr. Kingsley Sanders; then four months later I returned. I went into work every day and often on weekends, too, trying to get the feel of just what is involved in being a scientist pressing on a problem day after day. They were kind, hospitable and tolerant, tolerating not only my presence, but my leading, sometimes very personal, questions. In return, they made me a temporary member of the group, and this meant that intellectually no holds were barred. I was expected to understand what was being said, to grasp the direction of research, to defend my own arguments as if I had been in the game for a long time, and worst of all, to deliver a paper to their seminar on "Oesophageal Cancer Amongst the Turkomans." I missed Janez very much. So as we talked, discussed, observed and argued, I was whirled around in their eddy of activities, spun in a swirling vortex that was not self-contained or isolated, but interacted with a whole series of others. It is a good image, for the people and their ideas touch, bump and sometimes furiously collide with one another. The whole experience could have been interesting but no more, a stretch of time when, to use one scientist's phrase, we could have just gone "trickling along" through experiments, techniques, grant applications, seminars and the little local difficulties of culture contamination or the breakdown of apparatus.

As it happened, however, I stumbled in on them all during a most remarkable, unusual and then traumatic month. A vortex opened up, sucked me in, and a few weeks later spewed me out again, exhausted and battered. It was not only the effect of the human interactions and the scientific problems of the group, nor the heady euphoria of a real genuine discovery that propelled me. But I was inadvertently caught at the very center of the biggest scientific scandal of the decade, swirled round for two weeks in the vortex created by Bill Summerlin, having been with him the very day the issue broke. For many people at Sloan-Kettering, including me, things have never been quite the same since. (I deal with this episode in Chapter 7.)

To begin with, it was all deceptively ordinary.

I once asked Gip Wells, the son of H. G. Wells and himself a biologist, to give me a one-sentence characterization of a scientist. With his father's facility for quick thinking, he immediately came up with the following aphorism: "A scientist is a man who has the intellectual fidgets about the world." They are cerebral cats on conceptual hot tin roofs, and Kingsley Sanders, now fifty-seven, fits the description exactly. He is one of the most restless men I have ever met. He also talks incessantly, and by no stretch of the imagination could he be called beautiful. But his intellectual and physical restlessness catch the attention first. I have seen him in complete repose only three or four times, and the only sure way of capturing his attention fully is to talk compelling science. Even then the mind is ranging around; one can almost hear the firing of the neurons. He gives the impression of inhabiting a very private world. If he hasn't heard what you have said—and most of the time he hasn't—it is because most of his attention is focused on his internal conversation with himself. It is equally clear that he doesn't always hear or take in what *he* has just said, either. In the space of one hour he once told me the same story three times. When I came to think about this, I concluded that it really was because his mind is always following several strongly self-propelling directions. But he has the qualities of a born teacher, and this too stimulates the talk.

So from the time he bounced—he doesn't run or walk, but progresses by a speedy series of kangaroo hops—into the laboratory on that first Monday morning, all the activities of the next five weeks were conducted at a run. My mind immediately stretched on a mental rack: I had to strain every sense, not only to keep up with him, not only to get a word in edgeways, but also to assimilate and understand his thought.

With his colleagues Kingsley is wisely both much quieter and more attentive. I have seen him in meetings, both private and public, incredibly constrained, though one senses the fidgets underneath. When he speaks, he does so with intelligence and an assured authority. This quality of convinced assurance stems from his background: he was brought up in the confident atmosphere of Oxford at a time when there were still a number of eccentric polymaths around. No one single event propelled him into science; it was, he says, just the first thing he found that he could do well, among a host of other things he was interested in and enjoyed doing. The qualities of the polymath are still there, and science is just *one* of those things he enjoys doing: writing a novel is another, music a third. The present intense demands of science do not hold him strongly. Like one or two others I met during this work, he does not have that absolute, single-minded obsession with its hard core of toughness—roughness even. This inevitably affects the work he does and the rewards that he may expect.

His own scientific career can probably be characterized as a series of furiously active spurts involving some six or seven problems which have intrigued him. After he has worked a problem out to his own satisfaction, he admits that he goes into a phase of accidie, intellectual sloth, until another problem comes along that captures him. It is all very un-American and goes squarely against the Puritan ethic. But then he is very English indeed. He was in the zoology class of 1939 at Oxford that included such famous people as Sir Peter Medawar, amongst others. During the war he took his doctorate in neuro-histology and anatomy with J. Z. Young, and then switched his attention to viruses. In 1947 he came to America, to the U.S. Army's Walter Reed Hospital, which at that time was one of the few places giving a broad range of experience in experimental virology, then returned to Oxford, where he was able to set up a small laboratory in virology. Kingsley was one of the first people to realize that one could use animal viruses as probes to study the behavior of animal cells, as others had used bacterial viruses, phages, to study the behavior of bacteria. This was in the early 1950's, the exciting period that culminated in the famous Crick and Watson discovery, announced in 1953, of the structure of DNA. But when a senior colleague justified the squeeze on Kingsley's laboratory space with the astonishing statement that he couldn't see that the study of phages or the replication of nucleic acids held anything at all for the future of biology, Kingsley decided that he had to leave. Zoology at Oxford was to remain classical for some time.

So Kingsley joined the staff of the Medical Research Council; then in 1964 he received an award from the Sloan-Kettering Institute for a beautiful piece of work done with Montagnier showing how a single-stranded RNA virus could replicate. The Crick and Watson model suggested only how double-stranded molecules could replicate, but the single-stranded viruses were potentially embarrassing to the dogma. This work was Kingsley at his scientific peak as he followed a pattern of logic and method characteristic of good scientists: there is a specific question, so think and build a pyramid of induction. Then the experiment will suggest itself. Do it.

Later the Sloan-Kettering Institute tempted him over for a year's visit. After a two-year gap he returned to America again and has remained ever since. In this way cancer and viruses became his raison d'être, and in the weeks that followed, mine too, as I was piloted by this excitable, irreverent and self-absorbed scientist through a scientific maze. But before we began, he gave me two guides, one an aphorism and one a caution. "First," Kingsley told me, "this is a field where there is a specific goal, which is presumably the alleviation of cancer in man, but on the way there you'll get involved in the whole of biology. Second, in any laboratory the situation changes from day to day, and if you are to be any good, you must change with it."

I arrived at the Sloan-Kettering Institute on a Monday and for five days I stumbled around trying to get the hang of things. That Friday evening Kingsley and his wife, Irene, carried me off to Canaan in upper New York State, where they have a wonderful old house. We drove up in the dark and back in a blizzard, and that weekend was the first quiet chance to get some of the issues straight and to get clear about Kingsley's own ideas on viruses and cancer, and about the direction of the work. Saturday afternoon we sat in front of a log fire and argued, our discussion presided over by two beautiful brass candlesticks on the mantelpiece. They spiral in a helical manner and are known in the family as Crick and Watson. What emerged was this: work has now proceeded far enough for the question "Does this

cancer contain a virus or is it caused by a virus?" to be
meaningless. It is meaningless not because it is stupid, nor
because the relationship is unlikely, but because it leads to a
dead end. In order for any scientific question to have meaning, it
must contain within itself the elements for more questions and
more answers, so generating ideas and hypotheses and thereby
starting the chain of processes which will lead to testing by
experiment. In this sense it is no longer fruitful merely to see if
all cancers are caused by viruses, nor just to *find* the virus, in
those cases where the evidence is very strong. Scientists are now
one step further on; they are taking that small number of human
tumors which behave in such a way that viral involvement is
likely, working on those first and in depth, and trying to
determine the exact nature of the involvement and the exact
mechanism at work. They are searching, for instance, for the
watertight criteria which would enable them to say, "This virus
really does cause this cancer in human beings," or, "This is the
relationship between the state of malignancy in a cancer cell and
the incorporation of a virus." But, Kingsley emphasized, we
know so little at this point that we are in the primitive stage,
essentially the most creative stage in science. We only have the
sense of stumbling around in the dark, but this is the time
during which a hypothesis or a technique can come welling up
from the unconscious mind, triggered by a whole battery of
knowledge and past associations.

By now, I was beginning to realize that my notion of viruses
was wildly simplistic. First thing the following week I went to
talk to Alf Burness, another, younger, Englishman, who had
worked with Kingsley at the Medical Research Council, and
who also came over to Sloan-Kettering shortly after Kingsley
moved there. I had thought of viruses as small simple objects
like cherries, with a central core of genetic material and a soft
protein coat surrounding the core. However, they are much
more complicated than that. I also knew that they were in this
world simply to make more of themselves; they have no other
aim or end. In order to fulfill their destiny, however, they must
get inside a cell, and in order to do that, the protein coat must
slip off. We know that in some cases the virus latches onto a cell
and the protein coat dissolves away, allowing the genetic core to

slip in through the cytoplasm of the cell and eventually even into the nucleus, actually insinuating itself into the cell's genetic core. It is not particularly easy, for not only is the nucleic acid of all cells protected by the two barriers of cytoplasm and the nuclear membranes, but each molecule of nucleic acid is individually wrapped up in an ubiquitous shield of protective protein. But by some unknown mechanism, the virus slips through this last rampart, too, and is thus in position to take over the program of the cell. Now it can replicate and make more of itself. The process destroys the host cell, which bursts open, releasing new virus particles into the bloodstream; these go off to infect other cells. As the infection penetrates the body, the body's response mounts, and a sore throat and fever plus the routine of bed, fluids and aspirin usually follow. This is the simplest form of viral behavior, but other forms are quite viciously effective. One virus in one cell can do many things, depending upon whether a cell tolerates its presence or not, depending on what happens to the genetic material of the virus: whether the virus kills the cell as it grows within it, or whether it merely nestles down in a quiescent though potentially deadly embrace, quietly merging its own genetic component with that of its host. The virus may even do nothing at all . . . until later. There are certain viruses so deadly that they make the polio virus look positively benign. Scientists either no longer work with them or do so only in special laboratories under the conditions of the strictest care and caution, such as in Porton, England, or Frederick, Maryland.

All this Alf explained; then things began to get complicated. His office is decorated with models of viruses. There are diagrams on the bulletin board too, one of which is broken up like a jigsaw puzzle so that by reassembling triangles and squares, you can make your own "do-it-yourself germ" to order. What fascinates Alf is the relationship between virus structure and virus function. He puzzles over such questions as "What is it in the structure of the whole virus which gives it the character of a living thing? What is the structure of each little component? Exactly where is it in the virus and what does it do?" Viruses are not little balls but solid, regular and extremely complicated crystals. The outer shell of the Adeno virus, for example, is composed of 252 nut-shaped units, arranged in twenty equilateral triangles. Seen from the outside, the whole virus takes on the shape of an icosahedron.

I was fascinated to see that the regular solids have made a reappearance in science again after a period of some five hundred years. Their first appearance on the scientific stage came through Plato, who used shapes to explain the structure of atoms of air and fire, water and earth. Then Kepler utilized them, supposing that solid, regular structures filled the space between the heavenly spheres. Both men, it now appears, were looking at the wrong end of the universe. Regular solids occur now only in the minds of mathematicians and in the structure of crystals and the smallest particles of living matter. I asked Kingsley why this should be so; why shouldn't a virus have a completely irregular shape? He replied that possibly this was the only way to get a structure that could assemble itself, for a virus has the capacity not only of self-replication, but also of self-assembly. Taking it one step at a time, Alf took me through the structure and the classification of ten different viruses, describing the various pieces that have to be put together. By the time he had finished, my visions of cherries had vanished forever.

Alf works with a comparatively simple virus called EMC or encephalomyocarditis. It is not a glamour virus, nor is it dangerous, for, he confesses, he has no wish to be a hero. It is a kind of an Avis of a virus, number two. It is neither economically nor pathologically very important. "So why do you study this one?" I asked. "Because it tells us something very basic," he replied. It is as if I had come in to him and said, "Oh, by the way, how does a Rolls-Royce work?" And he had said, "Well, let's take a Model T Ford to bits first so we can get the basic principles, and then let's go on from there." Simple it may be, but it is also very remarkable. Hanging on the outside of the protein coat are various complicated bits and pieces from whose structure we can learn much, and whose function Alf is trying to assess. Inside, in the genetic core, there are coils and springs of genetic material just like the inside of a clock. Plato would have had a field day with it all.

Viruses behave in strange ways, in ways which explain why the virus particle does not show up in tumors except in rare cases.

The virus may penetrate the cell and be incorporated into the nucleus as part of the cell's genetic background. But then the cell may impose a strait jacket on the virus. So its genes are never expressed, and it cannot make its own proteins. The cell, however, can go on for a long time, happily ignoring the fact that there is a latent viral particle inside. Cells have superb mechanisms for controlling the expression of foreign genes. But there are also agents—some internal to the cell, some external— such as chemicals that are capable of removing the restraints. The viral genes can then be expressed, and if as a result they make a large quantity of viral proteins, as they do in a normal infection, the host cell may be destroyed. But if only a few viral proteins are made, they may just transform the cell. This seems to be the theory behind tumor formation by viruses. The covers come off of a small number of the virus genes. They then make a few proteins which are foreign to the cell, maybe as few as two, but these are enough to turn the cell cancerous. Only one or two genes of the virus may be at work, and one of the problems is to find out which these are.

We know that a virus can penetrate and remain quiescent for a very long time in human beings. The herpes virus that causes the familiar cold-sore blisters on the lip is a good example. There are many varieties. A herpes virus can infect the skin and a blister will break out; the cycle of infection will run its course, and apparently that is the end of the matter. But some time later—maybe months, maybe years—the infection will break out again. What has happened is that the viruses have insinuated themselves into the nerve endings, then moved up the fibers to a sensory ganglion just near the spinal cord. Here they stay quite passively until some sort of stress, such as sunlight or another trauma, even a mental one, triggers their activity once more. Then they pour down the nerve fiber and the pattern of infection begins again.

There was only one thing left to grasp, Alf told me. Essentially there are two types of virus; these differ only in the kind of nucleic acid inside. There are viruses of a particular form, roughly spherical, whose genetic core is of one form of nucleic acid, RNA. In animals, Type C viruses of this kind are known to cause leukaemia, a disease of the white blood cells, lymphomas, cancers of the lymph cells, and sarcomas, cancers of the muscles, cartilage and bone. The viruses of the famous herpes group, however, have DNA as their nucleic acid, and by now these have been suspected in a number of cancers in man; Hodgkin's disease, Burkitt's lymphoma, a childhood cancer first studied in Africa, and perhaps cervical cancer as well.

There are several basic difficulties which form an intellectual and technical barrier to answering the question "Do viruses cause cancer in humans?" One barrier is very obvious. The ultimate test is simply not possible; one cannot take a virus and inject it into human beings to see if tumors result. One must turn to models—animals—and from there extrapolate to the human situation. Immediately one confronts the second fundamental difficulty, one which occurs over and over again. Mice aren't men, nor is any other animal. So one question is very pertinent: Just what does an experiment with virus and tumor cells in a mouse *really* tell us about tumors in a human? The recent realization that we are also facing a species barrier has complicated this issue further. There are viruses which may cause only mild infections in one species, but when transplanted into another, cause a tumor. The owl monkey, for instance, carries a specific herpes virus within it quite happily, but if you inoculate marmosets with this virus, tumors result. The implications of this fact are rather unfortunate. You can extract a virus from human cells which you have reason to believe is implicated in human tumors, and you may inject it into a mouse and get a tumor, *but that fact alone* does not justify the conclusion that this virus will cause tumors in man. Since the ultimate test is impossible, what does one do?

There are three alternatives. You can try to see the virus in human tissue culture, try to "catch it in the act" at some stage in the tumor formation. Many cancers are very slow-growing: Hodgkin's disease is one of them. Though tumor viruses remain, we assume, in a close, repressed relationship with their host for a time, at some stage viral activity can be triggered in one cell. The cell then transforms, and as this occurs, the virus may reveal itself in some way or other. However, you can take millions of cells from the lymph nodes of patients with Hodgkin's disease, at all stages of the disease, and spend years looking at them under the microscope, and your odds on catching the one frozen instant of activity will be minuscule. So one must think of other ways to make the virus reveal itself.

Second, you can use your human material to get all the indirect evidence you can. The virus infections that cause epidemics have well-known patterns, so one can begin to search for suggestive epidemiological evidence. "Suggestive," not "convincing," for a disease like Hodgkin's disease, which may under certain circumstances be infectious, does not, thank heaven, affect many people. Because it is rare, one cannot get the kind of certainty that is necessary to be able to say unequivocally that there has been an infection. You can search for likely carriers, though, as a focus of infection, and then finally you can try to isolate the virus from the cells of patients.

Third, you can create a model system in animals—giving them Hodgkin's disease or something like it, and watching what happens—and you can also keep human tumor cells in culture, then put these cells into mice to see if they cause tumors. But you must also show that the virus can cause a tumor in the species of origin. That is, you have to demonstrate that the virus can cause human cells to be altered, but you must do this without risking a human life. Consequently, you try to "rescue" the virus. "Rescuing" the virus is a term in the trade for the various techniques which are used to capture the virus in some form or other. Once you have rescued the virus from one lot of human cells, you then infect other human cells in culture. If you can show that these newly infected human cells will now make tumors in mice with a higher frequency than uninfected human cells, you are almost home. Kingsley's group was trying to do this with regard to Hodgkin's disease, a cancerous disease of the lymph nodes. Because over many years it eventually spreads throughout the whole lymph system, it gradually depletes the body of those cells that resist infection, and then eventually the patient will die.

Their interest goes back to a study from upper New York State, done in the late 1960's, which suggested that "a smell of infectivity," to use Kingsley's phrase, hung around the pattern of Hodgkin's disease patients. That this should emerge at all seemed most unlikely, for this disease is very rare when compared with one like the flu, whose epidemic patterns obviously reflect the passage of a virus from person to person. But New York has had a cancer registry for a long time, so records existed as a source for possible clues. The scientists looked back at the pattern of Hodgkin's disease over several years and found a peak in 1954, followed by a trough; this pattern is a well-known feature of epidemics. So they went back to the cancer registry and pulled out all the cases of Hodgkin's disease at that time. Then, like Janez, they moved away from their desks and into the field, tracing the cases back to four students all in one high school in Albany at one time. Then they interviewed all the Hodgkin's disease cases for the following ten years, asking the patients whether they'd had any contact with the original group. Thirty-five patients had had either direct contact with the group or contact mediated by one other person. An individual is three times more likely to get the disease if he has a close relative who has it. These general epidemiological studies have been extended, and it seems possible that under certain circumstances Hodgkin's disease may be transmitted across the population; whatever is involved in the "infection," however, can remain latent and quiescent for a long time.

All this made the search for an infective agent a very reasonable enterprise, and the group, led by Kingsley and his colleague Dr. Magda Eisinger, went to work. The first difficulties were technical. The organ that might harbor the agent was clearly the lymph nodes of patients, so a technique had to be developed for growing a culture of human lymph node cells and for keeping them going for as long as possible. The group can now do this regularly, and the surgeons at Memorial Hospital just as regularly send down lymph nodes from Hodgkin's disease patients. Melna Hall, the technician responsible for the first stage, is warned ahead: the hospital calls immediately after an operation—generally early in the day. The node is stored in the appropriate medium and comes out to Rye from Manhattan on the 11:30 A.M. limousine, and Melna collects it. The next series of events can be completed within an hour, provided all goes smoothly, which it generally does. After washing several times, one piece is cut off and frozen for future reference. The remainder of the node is cut up very finely: part is put on

stainless steel grids to separate the cells; about fifty small pieces
are stuck down on tissue culture dishes; a great deal is macerated
for further tests; and one small part is shot straight onto slides
with a hypodermic syringe for immunological tests.

Starting and maintaining the cultures is the next step. The
cells are nurtured for a long time, feeding on a special medium,
and can be kept through a series of cell divisions. Long-term
tissue culture is a very delicate process. It is also a relatively new
technique for science, not done before 1950, and cancer research
depends on it very heavily. Amie Hemple, a senior research
technician with Kingsley, told me that it was like tending
delicate children. They have to be protected from infection and
fed a carefully controlled diet. By now there are standard recipes
for making up "cell food," as well as special diets for fastidious
cells. Some cells are, of course, more resilient than others, but
some, like Hodgkin's cells, are very fussy and discriminating
indeed. There is one very famous and tough line of human cells
called HeLa cells, taken from the cervical cancer of a woman
named Henrietta Lacks in 1951. These have taken to laboratory
conditions like a duck to water, and their descendent lines are in
a large number of laboratories all over the world. The cells are so
strong, however, that they are beginning to produce a situation
similar to what happened when rabbits were introduced to
Australia. If they contaminate another culture of more sensitive
cells, they first take over and dominate, then eliminate them.
Contamination of cultures is a standard scientific nightmare,
and the latest news on the cell-culture front is that many
commercial lines sold as pure cell lines of breast cancer tumors
or other human tumors and researched as such were thoroughly
contaminated with HeLa cells and were actually cervical cancer
cells all the time. This is truly a catastrophic situation, for a large
number of cultures must be thrown down the drain and a large
number of scientific results thrown away—many years of work
possibly lost. The cells can also catch bacterial infections or be
invaded by mysterious primitive microorganisms called mycoplasms. Whereas bacterial infections of cultures can be prevented with antibiotics, if mycoplasms contaminate the culture,
they can wreak total havoc and the culture then has to be
thrown out. It all adds up to a high degree of tender, loving and
very sterile care. Looking at the paper in *Nature* in which the

group announced some of their findings, I found an asterisk at one point, with a corresponding footnote that read: "Cell strain went through crisis at this time and expired." I sensed that the scientists also go through these crises "to the point of expiration."

After the cultures were successfully established, the group was able to go one step further in its search to identify and characterize an infective agent associated with Hodgkin's disease. They found that their cultures followed a common pattern. First there was an outgrowth of cells; then the cells went into a phase in which they resembled malignant cells taken from the late stages of Hodgkin's disease patients. For some unknown reason, in some cultures the cells would then lift off from the bottom of the flask, change shape and float. This happened fairly regularly, but most commonly the culture would go halfway through this process and stop. But in two instances all the cells transformed, and in both cases material containing labeled DNA and with the characteristics of a herpes virus appeared in the culture medium. And in one of those two instances they actually *saw* the herpes virus, and with the help of Dr. Etienne de Harven, an electromicroscopist, photographed it. Naturally they wrote a paper, which appeared in 1971 in *Nature*, that most prestigious scientific journal. With proper caution they reported "the recovery of virus-like particles from patients with Hodgkin's disease."

They've never managed to do it again; they've never seen the virus so clearly again, though they've been trying. For many reasons the dice are heavily loaded against them. In a disease that can spread out over thirty years, catching the frozen instant of viral activity involves a strong element of luck. So Dr. Eisinger began trying to get evidence from other directions, and on the very first day I met her, she apparently got it.

It came to be known as *Magda's Manic Day*, and that is how I shall always remember it. When I came to write about Magda, I knew I had to choose my words with care, for she is, without question, one of the most scrupulously honest persons I have ever met in my life. We came to know each other very well: I certainly learned a great deal from her and cherish the experiences of those weeks. The regret, if it comes at all, is anticipatory. If this one small thread of reluctance weaves into my recollections it is because I know how impossible it was, or will be, for me to measure up to that single-minded, golden honesty.

She came to America from Czechoslovakia in 1969, just after the Dubček debacle. She and her husband, Frank, were both in the universities and were very much for Dubček, but they are Jewish and have had some very bad experiences. One day she and Frank filled their car with their two daughters and their books and drove over the border to Vienna. It was after the Russians had come in, but just before the total clamp-down occurred, and to their great surprise, no one tried to stop them. Magda remembers this as a very poignant time, walking the streets of Vienna and being offered money by a Viennese to buy winter coats for her family. While they were in Austria, many Czechs came over to urge them to return. Eventually the situation became impossible, so they decided to come to America. When I met her early in 1974, her main concern was about her parents, who are both very old. Magda and Frank had been negotiating for months for them to come over for a visit, and this was a constant source of sadness and worry. Sadness, because it was hard on her parents to be left behind, never quite certain if retaliatory methods might be used against them. Worry, because being stretched out on the rack of expectation, even with regard to vacations, inevitably takes a toll. Four months later, however, on one hot September evening, I was to sit down to a goose and all the Czechoslovakian trimmings, with the whole family, parents included, in their New Jersey home.

I remember the "manic day" well. It was my second Tuesday and I came into the laboratory at eight-thirty in the morning. Kingsley had a meeting in town and wouldn't be in until noon. I was sharing Magda's office, a minute box off Kingsley's. It was wide enough for one desk and long enough for a desk and a half. Magda came in about nine o'clock. She had known that I was around and wanted to talk. In halting English she asked me to excuse her, perhaps for a half-hour. She had some experiments which had been going on all through the previous week and she wanted to look at the results, but when this was finished we would get together for a long talk. She was quiet and relaxed, charming and very polite, but clearly preoccupied. It was over an hour before she returned, and then she was flushed and very excited. She immediately apologized and began to stammer, "You see, something very exciting has happened . . . something very exciting. Come along and look." She took me to a small cubicle off Alf Burness's laboratory, where there is a fluorescence microscope. Dark curtains shut off the room so the only visible light came from the microscope, transmitted through the slide. She sat down, twirled a few knobs, and said, "Now look." I looked down the eyepiece and saw several small, brilliant spots, with the clarity of Sirius in the evening sky, shining like glowworms in the dark. The same phosphorescence can be seen on the shoreline, on a dark, warm, Mediterranean evening, when the waves are breaking. We went back to the office, and the look on Magda's face made me laugh. These intense spots of light were having the same effect as Joan of Arc's voices or Bernadette's visions, so I asked her to explain.

Like any thief viruses always leave their mark. We may not see them in action in tumors, but we see them easily in heavy infections. Sometimes we can surprise them; sometimes by "rescuing" techniques, we can force them to emerge, or at least force them to leave a fingerprint. I knew enough by then to know that catching the frozen instance of viral activity was very remote, but Magda *thinks* that after all this time, she may now have seen the "fingerprints" of the herpes virus possibly associated with Hodgkin's disease. Those italics are deliberate. One way to ruin our friendship forever would be for me to write those words assertively. She doesn't yet know, and while she doesn't, she would never forgive me or anyone else for saying or implying more. What seems to have happened is this:

Since the original experiment she has been trying to force the virus to reveal itself again. There are certain stages either in the progress of the disease or in the stages of the culture when this is probably easier to do than at any other time. The question was, How could she be certain of catching the virus activity, in a disease which might take over thirty years to run its course? The answer: possibly, only in tissue culture, just at the time when the cells are changing into the floating stage. This was the *only time* in their earlier experiments when they had found evidence of the genetic material from a herpes virus. It is now quite clear that during these stages the tumor cells produce several characteristic proteins of their own, and the virus inside the cells is also being forced to produce its protein. Magda suspects that in Hodgkin's disease they are dealing with a herpes virus, and therefore its antigenic expression, a herpes protein, was also being partially expressed in her cell lines. So she used the fluorescence technique on the cells to capture this expression. The spots of light she showed me were an indication of a reaction in which an antigen of the virus—a protein—reacted with a prepared blood serum. She had found her "fingerprint"—maybe.

Then she first used the word "beautiful" to me. It is one of her favorite words, and she uses it about anything which makes her really happy. "I have such beautiful projects, such beautiful problems," she says. "I am very lucky." By using "beautiful" in this context she means that there is such a simplicity about both the problems and questions that the answers are likely to be more or less clear-cut. With observations open to a variety of interpretations, ambiguity is a much more usual situation. Magda hates ambiguity, however, for she prefers not to have to speculate, if at all possible. Ultimately she wants to be able to say, "This *is* so." From this point of view, Hodgkin's disease is also a "beautiful" disease, because she has time. In a rapidly developing cancer, events pile up one after another, but in a situation where the patient moves slowly through four stages, the processes, whatever they may turn out to be, take longer; the events are spread out and *may* well prove easier to monitor. For Hodgkin's disease starts first of all with all the usual inflammatory infective reactions, perhaps the result of a "caught" infection. Then in the next stage, which is well separated in time, the virus possibly begins to transform the cells. Thus by choosing patients carefully from the Memorial Hospital clinic, one of the biggest Hodgkin's clinics in the whole world, Magda can hope to devise ways of following the virus through the four stages of Hodgkin's disease and observe through time the changing properties of those viruses which cause these tumors. On the other hand, the viral events may occur very rapidly, and she still won't catch the virus. We don't yet know. But the antigen she has revealed with this fluorescence may well be the expression of the DNA of the active virus, assumed to be associated with Hodgkin's disease.

She would like to see the virus, of course. This would be the best of all, so she has given samples of all the cells to the electron microscopists to see if they could *spot* the virus particles. Microscopists never jump to any conclusions, and all they would say at that stage was that they could see something "suspicious." So evidence from sight is lacking, but it seems to Magda that the sera taken from Hodgkin's patients at the early stages of the disease *are* indeed showing this particular Hodgkin's antigen, even though the sera from patients in the late stages of the disease are not. These later patients may be showing not the viral antigen, but several others—including an embryonic one, the F antigen, which, I was to learn, occurs over and over again in tumors.

Magda is very cautious indeed, but she does expect a virus to be somewhere around. She said she had been a little bit brainwashed before coming to America—she already believed that viruses were implicated in the causation of cancer. She was happy to work on Hodgkin's disease because it was a most "beautiful" model to look for possible virus cause. She was justified in calling the experiment "beautiful," for she had clearly caught the transforming process at a crucial moment. She was so thrilled that at one point I wasn't quite certain whether she was going to laugh or cry.

But what was so exciting about those fluorescent spots, and what was so "manic" about Magda? Her excitement came at several levels. Just as Magda had spotted the clue at a critical moment in time, so I too had spotted a scientist at a critical moment—the instant when she was trembling on the verge of something really significant. Without the virus, there can be no hope of a vaccine, of understanding its action or the course of a cancer; no hope of knowing which particular gene or group of genes is derepressed, so causing the cell to transform; no hope of understanding the infective pattern in Hodgkin's disease. We would never know whether the disease comes about because of one event, or whether there must be multiple "hits" on the cells. Even supposing we have the virus, of course—which we haven't, for we only have its "fingerprints"—there are many years of work ahead. Magda says that in those last five sentences, I have perhaps "jumped one hundred years of work." But this is a beginning, one more push forward, one more reason to suppose

that, in her own words, "In a few years we will really begin to
understand something of Hodgkin's disease."

The label "manic day" stuck, because at moments like these
Magda acquires some of the characteristics of an intellectual
and emotional hurricane. Her internal excitement spills over to
such an extent that it infects the people who work with her.
Moreover, her mood influences her work—not the results
themselves, of course, but the interpretation she is prepared to
put on them. I have noticed this with many other scientists, too.
One day Jack Hefton told me in a rush of amused affection,
"When Magda is having a 'manic day,' I choose that time to tell
her the results. On the days when she is up, a set of empirical
data are absolutely marvellous, 'beautiful.' But when she is down
she can find out everything, but everything, that is wrong with
the very same data."

There were other important aspects to the excitement. One
was the sheer human pleasure that comes in proving yourself
right and other people wrong, though Magda didn't put it to me
quite like that. When the group first discovered these viruslike
particles in Hodgkin's disease, many people thought they would
turn out to be the usual herpes virus, the Epstein-Barr virus, that
is implicated in Burkitt's lymphoma, and which seems ubiquitous. This isn't the case, however. The Epstein-Barr virus may
occur in almost every normal human being, but not in the lymph
nodes of Hodgkin's disease patients, Magda says. Her studies
show that her specific antigen is totally negative to the standard
E.B.V. antibody, and is quite specifically itself a variant of
herpes.

A second aspect is that there could be some exciting
therapeutic possibilities from these experiments, and here the
slow progression of Hodgkin's disease would help us. The virus is
first expressed at the beginning of the tissue culture in the form
of the nuclear antigen. Then much later the cells produce a
second cytoplasmic antigen, and then later a third, if not more.
These antigens probably mask the real situation, because
patients at stage three and four may be making antibodies not
against the virus, but against other antigens. That doesn't help
them at all, for it is then too late. So if one is going to knock out
Hodgkin's disease, Magda's research may tell that you *must* do

so in the early stages of the disease, if at all, before the deceptive antigens are called into play.

We talked that morning for three hours, and at one point Magda said, "I don't want to tell Kingsley yet, because he will get so excited." I found this hilarious, considering the state she was in, and asked why not? What would happen if he got excited? "When this happens," she said, "he turns in so many directions at once that I cannot follow." She kept her resolution for precisely one hour. When Kingsley returned from his meeting, I invited them both out to lunch, and somewhere between the soup and the sea bass, she broke her resolution. Trying to keep it all in was like trying to push the cork back into a bottle of champagne at the very moment of opening. Kingsley took it very calmly indeed. This was one of his moments of repose, and for an hour I sat and listened, interjecting very little, as the two scientists considered the implications together.

I was watching two people with distinct personalities, distinct ambitions, interacting together as they focused on one scientific problem. What they would claim, how they would proceed, how they would even conceive the problem, differed in certain substantial respects. The people they are does affect the science they do. Their disagreements should not surprise us, although the conflicts can sometimes become so great that the tensions become intolerable and a parting of the ways inevitable. The source of real strength in scientific collaboration, however, often lies in the degree of creative conflict between the participants: the Crick-Watson collaboration, where the two participants deliberately chose to disagree, is a case in point. No scientist really likes to collaborate, and if they all had adequate funds, adequate space and adequate time, they would work alone. As Magda told me, "We are all in little private boxes. Each of us thinks his or her problem is *the* most important problem and that he or she is doing it in the most important way."

The differences and the conflicts between Magda and Kingsley emerged the moment I began to question them about the real meaning behind the 1971 paper. What did they really think the results meant, and what had they been doing since then? Both of them agreed on one thing: the results gave evidence of a herpes involvement in Hodgkin's disease, but not proof. There has still been no definite evidence from other people either, though Dr. Zamecnik and his team in Boston have produced some corroborative immunological support. But large gaps remain. Given the initial results, other people in other laboratories might well have moved fast and furiously to nail the evidence down. For the question still remains: What was it they saw? Was it truly a viral particle associated with or implicated in Hodgkin's disease, or just a viral cell product thrown up by their procedures? In order to nail this issue they should, if possible, have gone on to demonstrate some relation of that particle to viruses known to be associated with human cancer.

But Magda's personal quest for the Hodgkin's disease agent is being conducted in her own highly distinctive and cautionary style. She proceeds step by step, following out one line or one consequence very carefully, never moving on until she is totally secure in her experimental footholds. The pace and the logic are obvious to her: it is the only way to work. She had hoped to see the virus particle again; since she did not, she used immunological tricks to make it betray itself. She thinks she now has done this and has caught the viral protein. Now she must see whether this antigen can be found in all cultured cells from Hodgkin's disease patients, not just from transformed cells, and whether it corresponds to any other known viral antigen. She might have to devise other techniques, too, to "rescue" the virus: perhaps the highly dangerous ones of hybridization, which involve "marrying" a part of one virus with part of another to produce a viral "bastard." Since we have absolutely no idea of the properties of these bastards, whether they will be benign or vicious, such experiments present a real biohazard. Consequently, Magda would either have to go to Fort Detrick or wait until fully protective laboratories are available at Rye. In either case she will develop her experiments in a careful sequence, eliminating all ambiguity. She will not commit her ideas to paper or convert her private thoughts into public words until she is "quite sure."

In this way she reveals both her strengths as a scientist and her weaknesses. For how "sure" is "sure"? How certain should you be before you take a stand, and how many times must you do an experiment or a variation on it before the possibility that you may be wrong is totally eliminated? The race to publish, and publish fast, in American science is reflected in the well-known aphorism "Don't get it right, get it written." But in her anxiety to be right, Magda runs the risk of never writing. She takes her time over publication, and this dismays many of her colleagues who admire her work. The caution and her demand for total certainty may have roots in her past. But she is an unforgiving person, and she will tolerate divergence from the truth in no one—especially in herself. The core of her science is the core of her being.

I was not surprised, therefore, by the answer I received when I said, "What may I quote as your considered opinion on the results described in your *Nature* paper and their significance?" She took about five minutes to answer, thinking the words out very carefully in an agonized torture of cerebral labor. Then she said, "The supernatant fluid of cells labeled with DNA precursors [the building blocks of DNA], and assayed for the presence of particles containing DNA in sucrose-density gradients, showed the presence of this labeled material in an area where *some* DNA viruses could band. When the bands were presented with antisera against a herpes virus, they gave a positive reaction." I asked her to be more informal. She said, "The work was an introduction only. It showed us ways to grow cells from the lymph nodes of Hodgkin's disease patients in culture, so now they can be studied in more detail. The results also pointed to the presence of herpes antigen in these cells." Just a few sentences. To say any more would be mere hypothesis, and while she might think hypothetically, she will not speak so. She is keeping her imagination on the tightest of reins, and only time will tell how detrimental this will be to her scientific career. She will not commit herself and gets furious with anyone else who leaps ahead. Of course, this means that from time to time she gets incensed with Kingsley, who could no more tolerate a moratorium on unexpressed hypothesis or unfettered imaginative excursions than he could on speech. He would suffocate. So when I asked him the same question I received not two sentences, but two hundred. He immediately embarked on a wide-ranging scientific jaunt setting the specific details of their experiment into a number of general frameworks of disease, of infective patterns, of cancer, of biology. The evidence for his statements varied from utterly solid to the completely tenuous as he spun off possibilities that will demand years of experiment to confirm.

He believes that they did get a herpes virus and that this *possibly* was the infective agent in Hodgkin's disease. Different specific antigens do appear in the cultures which *are* unique herpes antigens, and there might be other viruses at work here. But even if their particular virus particle was *the* infective agent, they would still have to explain how this agent could cause such a "rare" disease. The evidence from animals tells us nothing about how human tumor-causing viruses might be passed on. So, Kingsley went on, we must continue the laboratory work on human material, and also be theoretical, trying to construct hypotheses both for the causes of Hodgkin's disease and for its transmission. We must work out a model system in animals from which we can extrapolate back to the human situation. Above all, we must sharpen our criteria for proof. Kingsley can hope to do only a small fraction of what his thoughts imply.

Listening to them both one day, I wondered whether if I took the best qualities from each and made a hybrid scientist, much as they make a hybrid virus, would this person be highly successful? It is most unlikely. Their respective traits are so contradictory that the hybrid would probably be in a perpetual state of scientific schizophrenia. It would be like marrying Agatha Christie's Miss Marple to G. K. Chesterton's Father Brown, and expecting the resulting detective to solve all mysteries instantly. And there would be no guarantee that the scientific sleuth would function, for too many elements would be at war with each other. Her single-minded persistence, puritanical belief in prolonged hard work, bewilderment at, and even marginal disapproval of, such frivolous activities as novel-writing, could not coexist with his relaxed irony and deliberate cloak of irreverence, even while she might admire his wide background and consciously cultivated knowledge. They are best as they are—two separate, real, people—and scientifically they are now going their separate ways.

These last five years have transformed Magda. The collaboration produced more than just a paper in *Nature*. "Kingsley forced me to become independent," she says. "It was traumatic. But the experience wasn't valuable just for that. It was important for my confidence, for he doesn't tell you what to do. He lets you work on what interests you—and this is very unusual—and good." Secure in the background of her new life in America and confident of herself as a good scientist, Magda is now striking out on her own independent line, obstinately doing her science in precisely her own way. My guess is that as her career develops, so, too, will her imagination be liberated. In any case, she has achieved something else really significant.

The first authenticated human tumor-causing virus to be cultured indefinitely and fully described may come from her laboratory. First details may have been published by the time this book is out. The lucky girl has not one, but two "beautiful" problems. The second one is warts. I knew nothing about warts, but they, too, are tumors and are caused by viruses. They are benign tumors; in a wart the virus behaves in a manner halfway between its behavior in an infection and its behavior in cancer. They are therefore very important to study.

When you get a wart, it means that one cell has become infected by a virus, and eventually a benign tumor is produced. The tumor never spreads, never metastasizes and will go away. The only exceptions are in patients whose immune system has been suppressed either by disease or drugs; in these cases the warts *never* go away. But the lethal potential remains, especially if the viruses cross the species barrier. One kind of wart virus causes benign tumors in wild cottontail rabbits, but malignant tumors in domestic rabbits. The colony effect—the cloning—of a cancer is seen very beautifully in a wart. A cell in the lower layer of the skin becomes infected and divides very rapidly. It may well be that several cells become infected, but the cellular environment around the wart is such that one population wins over all the others. The probable sequence of events is as follows, though, as Magda insists, there is no tight evidence for this process. The virus goes through only half its life cycle. It doesn't produce more of itself, so the cell does not burst open. Instead, it causes the cell to transform partly, but no more virus is produced. But if the viral life cycle is completed, the wart vanishes, because the accumulative result of that virus production stimulates a pathogenic effect, just like in an infection, and the body responds to it. If this sequence proves to be generally true of all viruses, our best technique against cancer might be to make the *viruses replicate* somehow, and complete their life cycle.

It is not to the virus's advantage to form a tumor since its object in life is replication, and when it produces a wart, this object is defeated. What stops the virus from replicating? It may well be that we do, and it is most unfortunate. It may be that our responses to a minor infection are as minor as the infection itself. We react a little, perhaps just enough to stop the virus from completing its cycle, and the price we pay for this is a tumor. "What stops the virus going through its cycle?" I had asked Kingsley. "Well," he replied, "the herpes virus may not be in the right cell, it may not be in the right environment." Scientists talk of "susceptible" and "nonsusceptible" tissues, or "permissive" and "nonpermissive" cells. In a nonsusceptible tissue, the virus never gets in; but sometimes a cell can become "permissive" to a virus, and the virus replicates inside it. Kingsley said several times, "If only we could get the virus to replicate," and I completed the statement: "We wouldn't get a tumor."

Kingsley also often said, "If Hodgkin's disease is an infection, then the agent has to complete its cycle somewhere." How else could it be transmitted to another person? He suspects that in this disease the virus may replicate somewhere in the oral cavity. In the case of wart viruses, the agent passes from cell to cell only by contact, not by floating in the air, and the virus sometimes does complete the cycle in the very cells where it began. Then the body responds and defeats it. But if the cycle is not completed, a benign tumor results. Warts, then, give us a whole spectrum of viral activity, with consequences that are sometimes mild, sometimes malignant. It has been known for some time that they were caused by a virus, *papovavirus*, but neither the life history nor the structure of this virus has ever been fully described because no one had been able to culture it in quantity. Magda has now become the first person to do this. She can keep the virus going—not only in one cell line, but for at least twelve passages in culture. (This means she can infect a cell, recover the virus, infect another cell, recover the virus, infect another cell, and so on.) Though other people have tried, no one else has succeeded in this before, and she now does it with such facility that when I asked her, "Why did other people fail?" she answered, "I can't possibly imagine."

She had first tried all the known techniques. If scientists published their negative results—as well as their positive ones—

it would, Magda insists, save everyone a lot of time, energy and money. Since they don't, she had to go through the whole gamut of failure herself. A human cell line derived from skin had been established by Dr. Mike Bean, and in this she tried to culture the wart virus, using all the known dietary blandishments and environmental encouragements. She calls this "The Story of My Non-Think Tank." Day after day, week after week, they tried, yet the virus wouldn't "take" or survive in this cell line. Then one day, to her astonishment, it worked beautifully. So she and her technician Olga, also from Czechoslovakia, asked themselves, "What did we do this time that was so special, so clever?" The answer was "Absolutely nothing!" It turned out that overnight there had been a cylinder failure. The carbon dioxide tank, which supplied the gaseous background to the cells, had run out, and the chemical background for the cells changed—for the better, as far as the *papovavirus* was concerned. By accident she learned that by monitoring and adjusting the acidity of her culture, she could recover the virus in vast quantity. They now have electron microphotographs of the wart virus, and she will now start to characterize it. The structural description has been done, but not the molecular biology nor the life cycle. The possibilities that now open up are exciting for clinicians as well as virologists. They can at last try to develop a vaccine, and this will be useful for people with multiple warts, whether they arise from mere infection or from some deficiency in the immune system. Magda can extend the work on the viral proteins produced in human warts and in carcinomas of the skin. She can then look at the immunological questions: why do warts sometimes go away and sometimes not, and does this bear any relationship to the activity of the virus in the cell? She might also be able to set up a model system which would answer such quantitative questions as how much virus is needed for one given lesion, and how many lesions are produced from a given quantity of virus. She has plenty to keep her busy.

As the days went by in this one small corner of the scientific world, I rapidly came to realize that the days of simplistic views are over. Peyton Rous started a chain of work with what appeared to be a simple cause-effect description: a virus makes a tumor. It is infinitely more complicated than that—just how complicated we can hardly conceive. J. B. S. Haldane, a great biologist, once said, "The world is much queerer than we realise; in fact, I think it is queerer than we *can* realise," and as I stayed at Sloan-Kettering, I saw just what he meant. In recollection, my mental pictures of those days are as crowded as the laboratories. I tuned in very quickly to the private "in" jokes, seeing the cartoons on the walls as an expression of the current problems in science. If I really thought to interpret them in this way, then the cut in funds is the area of greatest concern. There is the unshaven, disheveled man sitting on the pavement outside Capitol Hill, with his upturned hat on the sidewalk and a placard across his chest saying *Grantless*; or two drunk scientists in a downtown bar, steeped in a maudlin alcoholic haze, and one of them saying, "Ninety percent of scientists who ever lived are alive today." The other replies, "Yes, and twenty percent of them are out of work."

I soon came to appreciate the force of those little-known, but very pertinent scientific principles. "No amount of planning will ever replace dumb luck!" said a notice in the seminar room. Murphy's Law: "If anything can go wrong, it will"; Cahn's Axiom: "When all else fails, read the instructions"; Horner's Five Thumb Postulate: "Experience varies directly with the equipment ruined." These are all true, but the Rule of Accuracy has the quality of an eternal verity: "When working towards the solution of a problem, it always helps if you know the answer." The Advanced Corollary reads: "Provided, of course, that you know there is a problem." Viruses and cancer together make a real problem.

As an outsider, with neither their motivation nor their sense of urgency, I wondered afterwards what it was that saved those days from turning into a scientist's article in a learned journal, objective and detached, and therefore to a writer, potentially uninteresting. Except for the localized excitement of Magda's Manic Day, there was no beating of brows or of breasts; I heard no shrieks of "Eureka!" as world-shattering discoveries poured forth. It was mostly a very low-key operation, but the interplay of people and their problems—scientific, personal and political —was continually interesting, with a combination of zest and enthusiasm, frustration and irritation, joshing and anger, all of which together with creative ideas adds up to science as it is practiced. The outside world is never far away, however, and this activity has to be both justified and examined.

At the end of my first week, the Board of Scientific Consultants came to pay a visit. This important procedure takes place twice a year: a band of extremely distinguished scientists visits various sections of the institute to discuss problems, intellectual and logistical, with scientists of the various laboratories in turn. Then they have a very private meeting with the director and associate director, to voice their criticisms and make their recommendations. I sat in on the first part of the procedure. One doesn't need a Royal Family to generate the feeling of a State Occasion. The windows in the main hall were washed. A most beautiful new ceiling had been quickly installed into a newly converted room across the corridor. Stuart Marcus (see Chapter 3) came to work clean-shaven that day, and Kingsley even tidied his desk—by the simple expedient, I believe, of opening the drawers and shoving everything inside. He also wore a suit, but he swore that it had nothing to do with the occasion. He had started the morning in his usual slacks and jacket, but had been caught in a sudden downpour while exercising the dogs and so had to change. We didn't know whether to believe him.

The Royal Family analogy is indeed a good one, for the institution of the board resembles that of the constitutional monarchy, with all the trappings, but none of the power. The board can neither hire nor fire; it cannot take away grants or bestow favors. Their role is advisory only, and the extent of even that depends on the inclination of the director, Dr. Robert Good. His immediate predecessor, Dr. Frank Horsfall, never acted without taking advice, and while it is clear that the present director has a streak of independence, it is equally clear that he uses his consultants extensively as critical hones on which he, as well as his colleagues, are required to sharpen up their ideas. Thus while the repercussions from the views of members of the board may be limited, pregnant possibilities *do* exist, so there was, I felt, an unmistakable quality of tension in the meetings, especially on the part of the younger scientists. This band of consultants, led now by Sir Peter Medawar as chairman, are very bright indeed, and the direction of a scientist's work, or the effort eventually put behind it, may well be influenced by their recommendations. One of the issues, among many others, brought before the board arose after presentations by Kingsley and Magda. The scientists argued that a biohazard facility should be built at Rye so that they could move on to the next stage of their experiments, which would include viral hybridization. During the discussion the issue turned, I recall, not on the necessity of the facility as such, for everyone agreed that whenever such experiments are done containment facilities are vital. But the question focused more on a question of principle: Is the situation in viral research now at the stage where *all* such experiments were best conducted at government institutions such as Fort Detrick? When I returned to the Sloan-Kettering Institute a few months later, I heard that a biohazard facility was to be constructed, so I infer that the board did in fact recommend this.

But eventually the State Occasion was over and things reverted to normal. The very next day Kingsley's desk was as chaotic as ever, and as if to celebrate the relaxation of tension, the ceiling in the new laboratory fell down at once. My novelist's mind went to work: under the pile of plastic debris there was a dead virologist, killed with a lethal virus by a colleague, who then promptly autoclaved the evidence away. Then Kingsley went up to Canaan for eight days. It was Irene's midterm vacation, and he had a grant application to write. But he must have taken a virus with him, for over the telephone both he and Irene sounded dreadful. The virus was replicating, all right: they had massive infections. So he was not around at the time of crisis and distress, that aberrant moment of the Summerlin affair when the possibility had to be faced that a scientist in another part of the institute had willfully misrepresented his data. Though it was some weeks before most people knew just what had occurred, the atmosphere was restless and uncertain. So it was a relief when Kingsley finally returned from the country and Magda came out to Rye again from Manhattan, providing me with indexes of solid scientific security.

Suddenly there was a moment when everyone, or nearly everyone, was in the same room. We knew that people were around that day, and perhaps for no other reason than that the others had so many questions and queries for Kingsley and Magda, it just happened that we all gravitated together. For one of those small, frozen instances, the time it takes to see a virus or to form an impression, the group was all smiling, immensely pleased to see one another. Then the moment dissolved, and the vortex caught them up. The impressions of affection would later dissipate, to be replaced for a time by tensions and conflict, to be replaced again by warmth. For the human relationships expressed by the group are no more immutable than the scientific problems which hold them together. One can be damaged by viruses and by personalities, but one can also be bound, and all scientific groups experience this.

The Sunday before I left I spent the whole day in the office, working over my notes, letting the layers of comprehension gently settle in my mind. As I walked down the corridors, classical music was pouring from the radio that the security guard had in the hall. I knew I was going to miss the place, even those horrible torsos, the plastic germ-free isolators that the scientists use as sterile containing devices to manipulate their viruses in safety. Kingsley is convinced that when the doors close in the evening and the scientists go home, these torsos roll down the corridors and take over. My theory is that they stay in their rooms, and in collaboration with the viruses do experiments on the torsos of scientists who have been knocked unconscious when the ceilings have fallen down!

So what gives? as Bernie often said to me. We don't know yet. But before I left, Kingsley summed up the present state of the art: "There is no clear picture. All human cells may contain some viral genes; we are pretty certain of this. Under unknown circumstances, which may be another virus or a chemical influence, the virus may be expressed, and this may cause cancer. One trick will be to find the circumstances that produce this, but if we do, it may tell us nothing about the natural etiology of the disease. By various manipulative tricks, we can probably study the degrees of expression of these viruses, and possibly relate this to malignancy. We *know* that this work is going to be important for biology, for we shall learn a great deal about these entities. But as for its importance for cancer, we don't yet know, for the initial viral event that leads to a tumor probably takes place very quickly indeed."

We in society, however, have our expectations, and the first word one associates with viruses is "vaccines." It is a long time since the days of Jenner and smallpox vaccine. In theory, it is just possible that we may produce cancer vaccines, but in practice we must be honest and admit that it is a very long way away. The properties of the virus dictate what we can or cannot do with them. For a start, we cannot vaccinate against those viruses which are transmitted vertically from mother to child. In those cases the child is born already infected, already tolerating the virus, so nothing can induce the child to make antibodies. This rules out vaccines against those viruses like leukaemia virus which we believe may remain hidden in the body and may be passed on through generations. Viruses like herpes, on the other hand—which, since we catch them from other people, are transmitted horizontally—would seem to present a more suitable case for treatment. But even here there are difficulties, for herpes is ubiquitous and comes in a variety of forms. And if it settles in the nerves, away from the blood, it cannot be reached by any circulating antibodies. Any human cancer virus of the herpes type may well have this same property, being so deeply associated with its host that we may never reach it.

In addition, no vaccine has ever been made which is effective against any herpes virus in man, though new reports from Germany do claim a successful vaccine against *Herpes simplex*. But even if we have a successful herpes vaccine, we could not give it to a newborn baby. We have something better to do with them than inject them against the possibility of Hodgkin's disease at the age of twenty. It is such a rare disease that mass vaccination would not be worthwhile; we would want to vaccinate only a high-risk group. But the immunological system is not functioning until the child is three months old, by which time that ubiquitous herpes is all around, if not already ingrained in the body.

So we may be forced to concentrate on other forms of immunological attack on cancer viruses, or we may have to figure out how to exploit those reactions of our immune system which already counter them. One type of attack would be to stimulate the lymphocytes, help those cells in their "creative" process of eating up viruses. Indeed, as this book is being written, Dr. Stanley Order reports that he and his colleagues at Harvard have made an antibody against one of the antigens associated with Hodgkin's disease. The antigen, a ferritin compound, is ubiquitous, and is found in many tumors as well as in embryonic tissues. The antibody was given to a volunteer patient with advanced recurrent Hodgkin's disease, and it homed directly onto the tumor masses, where it remained for eight days. This work is part of the continuing search for "lethal therapeutic packages" which may eventually be delivered precisely and specifically to a tumor.

Moreover after viral infections, animal cells can release a substance, interferon, which serves as a general attacking agent against all viruses. It sometimes also seems to have the property of seeking out and destroying cancer cells. Although complete cures have not yet been reported, it can be effective against even quite large tumors, although here the sudden destruction of large numbers of tumor cells may release substances that poison the system. Interferon's supreme advantage is that, compared with other anti-tumor substances, it is entirely without toxicity. So that although enormous amounts may be needed to treat human tumors effectively, this may be an incentive to their production.

So why study viruses if we cannot vaccinate against them? Because they may be the most important scientific weapon we possess for this battle. We *must* find the precise differences between a normal and a malignant cell. We must understand the mechanism of the transformation from normal to malignant and the results of the change. Perhaps one viral protein alone, the expression of just one viral gene, may be the lethal unit that will give us the vital clues to this understanding. Viruses are our guide through the maze of cell malignancy. They are both the nastiest problem in biology *and* the tool to solve it.

3

CANCER AND BIOLOGY:
A PRICE WE PAY FOR LIFE

A comprehensive and penetrating understanding of the molecular and biological nature of cancer is very near at hand, so near that when we look back four or five years from now it may be difficult to say which discoveries were most important in gaining this understanding.

—Professor van Rensselaer Potter, speaking
at the Princess Takematsu Symposium on
Cancer Research, Tokyo, 1973

THE DISCOVERIES are pouring in, raining down thick and fast in a positive deluge of empirical data. If we don't yet understand the nature of cancer and the transformation from a normal cell to a cancerous cell, it is not for want of trying. But to concentrate only on the data is to take a very limited view of the word "discovery." In any case, empirical data alone are not going to help us achieve our goal. In order to devise a rational therapy of cancer, in order to *comprehend* prevention, diagnosis and prognosis as well as treatment, we are going to have to construct a general theory. We shall have to impose a pattern on the accumulated facts. We should not expect too much, however. Maybe in the end the only thing that a general theory will do for us is give us great intellectual satisfaction. Maybe a theory that explains cancer in terms of evolution and molecular biology and the unbelievable complexity of the cell will in the end show us only why we cannot do what we would like to do. It may also tell us why we never will totally eliminate cancer; why the causes can never be totally eradicated; why we are unlikely to spot a cancer at its inception.

Early in this work I concluded that scientists are not easily embarrassed, for the three main causes of cancer—chemicals, viruses and radiation—have been known as such for years. Remembering how many doctors and scientists have already brought their minds to bear on this subject, one could perhaps be justified in asking, "What have they been doing all this time?" But if scientists are not easily embarrassed, they are right to remain unruffled. For they appreciate that the majority of us outside the profession do not even understand—namely, that one very important concept in science is the concept of "unripe time." One discovery does indeed wait upon another. Sir Peter Medawar's aphorism "Science is the art of the soluble" not only holds in cancer as in every other field of science, but illustrates it better than any other I know. What he meant was not so much that science is the "art of solving problems" but that it is the "art of solving problems which can be solved"—that is, which are ripe for solution. A good scientist is only one or two steps ahead, not twenty, for theoretical problems will yield only when the knowledge, the techniques and the tools are all at hand to solve them. There may be many scientists who feel that given our present knowledge, the effort in cancer *is* disproportionate and premature, since the intellectual challenge is being mounted too soon. This may or may not be so, but before 1953 would certainly have been far too soon, for our knowledge of the gene is only some twenty years old.

To understand cancer, one must first understand all over again the nature of heredity. The end products of cancer, tumors and metastasizing cells, result from the piling up of a series of catastrophic events. Given a fundamental change in hereditary make-up, whether caused by a virus or a chemical, the cell begins to breed true, forming a colony of cells with a formidable battery of altered properties. At heart, then, the problem of cancer is a problem of inheritance and the control mechanisms of a cell, and this forces one back to the basic molecules of life, DNA and RNA. Lord Ritchie Calder recounts with pleasure how as a reporter on the *Daily Express*, he convinced his editor to lead off an article with "Deoxyribonucleic acid. Deoxyribonucleic acid. Deoxyribonucleic acid. Repeat it. Spell it and repeat it again. It is the most important word you will ever have to learn." It was a most telling index of importance.

There are plenty of books giving beautiful accounts of the molecule, its discovery, structure and properties: James Watson's *The Double Helix,* Jacques Monod's *Chance and Necessity,* John Maddox's *Revolution in Biology.* It is easy to make a model yourself. All you need to do is make a long paper ladder, anchor the bottom ends with Scotch tape, hold the top ends in one hand and apply a gentle twist in an anticlockwise direction. This model of the molecule then immediately takes the shape of the molecule—the double helix. The sides of the twisted ladder reflect the spiral phosphate backbone of the molecule. If before twisting the paper ladder, you put two dots in the middle of each rung, the model then takes on something of the finer structure. On each rung of the ladder are two chemical bases, held together by a light chemical bond of hydrogen. These bases go in matching pairs, so if you use different colored dots to represent different bases [blue, adenine (A); red, thymine (T); green, guanine (G), yellow, cytosine (C)], wherever you put a blue dot, say, a red one must be painted opposite it and on the same rung; in the same way, a green one must go with yellow. In other words, if there is adenine on one rung, the other half of that rung always has thymine, and a sequence running up one side of the ladder reading A.T.C.G. *must* mean that on the opposite side the sequence will run T.A.G.C.

To be really sophisticated, after having placed the bases, you should split up the center of each rung, and with the lightest of wire threads join the bases up again. These threads would represent the hydrogen bonds, which can break easily. They *must* break, for this molecule has two important properties: it makes more of itself and it provides the template for a process whose end result is protein.

To make more of itself, the DNA molecule begins to unzip from one end, and the DNA precursors, the bases which are being synthesized in the cell cytoplasm, come up as matching chemicals, in their corresponding order, to build a new strand opposite each half. Where there is an adenine base on the half-thread, a thymine will be brought in to pair opposite it;

opposite a guanine base, a cytosine will be set. The phosphate backbone will be attached to the sequence of bases, and ultimately there will be four strands of matching DNA where at first there were only two. Once this process of self-replication has been completed in the nucleus, the cell can divide.

All cells start from the same single fertilized egg, which has been given a complement of male and female chromosomes— twenty-three from the mother and twenty-three from the father. So in the beginning of an individual's life cycle, there is one common unit of genetic material: an array of DNA molecules, functioning genes strung out along the forty-six chromosomes. But if all cells start with the same complement of DNA, what makes adult cells different from each other—a liver cell with its characteristics of a chemical-processing factory, a muscle cell with its capacity to contract? The answer is protein.

Protein-making occurs in two stages, transcription and translation. A transfer of information takes place in the same way that the information in my head is dictated onto a tape in one form of words, which reappears in this book as another form of words. Words as thoughts become words as electrochemical impulses become words in print. Similarly, in the first phase of protein-making, transcription, the information from one form of nucleic acid, DNA, is turned into information in another form, RNA, a similar acid but with one of the bases different. The RNA molecule moves around the cytoplasm, carrying the information needed to specify the proteins that the adult cell must make in quantity.

As the cell progressively matures, the genes are switched off in turn. In a fully functioning muscle cell, for example, with its characteristic protein, myoglobin, only one or two genes will be left operating. The rest will have been repressed. It has been estimated that in an adult cell only 0.001 percent of the DNA is transcribed, for by the time a cell is fully differentiated most of it is permanently shut down. Only that portion of the DNA whose bases code for the correct proteins will be in action. The messenger RNA, matching up to the appropriate part of the DNA, takes the information for this protein as a sequence of bases to the protein power plant in the cell. Meanwhile, another form of RNA is scavenging around, assembling the various amino acids which will be necessary to build the particular protein molecule required. The correct sequence is read off the messenger RNA and the building blocks are assembled in correct order, just as the compositor of this book read the words of my manuscript and assembled the letters to make up my words and sentences. What began as a thought in my head ends as the printed word. What begins in the DNA ends as a protein, by the processes of transcription and translation. All this is under very precise control of the biological catalysts, enzymes, which speed up or slow down the process. Without enzymes there would be no protein synthesis: without DNA there would be nothing.

DNA, then, is the basic material for life, the matrix for evolution. It is found throughout the living world, differing in amount and size but not differing one iota in general structure. The order of the four bases codes for every protein we know; the material can at one and the same time specify an amoeba, a mouse or a man. Without its structure it must maintain a most delicate balance between two conflicting properties. The DNA must be stable; this is why it is hidden away in the nucleus surrounded by protein, protected from those environmental changes that might alter it. Yet on the other hand, the molecule must not be so stable it never changes at all. It must be capable of variation, and of variation that persists. Many of the paradoxes of life have arisen from the conflict between these two apparently mutually exclusive properties. There must be subtle changes in the DNA, because otherwise all children would be like their parents. All cells born of the primordial cell would be identical with it, and natural selection would have nothing on which to work. But the changes must not· be so drastic as to be damaging to the embryo. For then there would be no offspring at all. Yet what happened during evolutionary time? An infinite variety of remarkable living forms evolved, culminating in the most subtle and complicated organism of all, composed of millions of cells. Each cell in its internal workings is a network of processes almost as complicated as the organism itself. Now if one begins to think about cancer against this background, contradictions spring up like weeds in spring. If cancer is so lethal, why is it still around? Why in the course of evolution have we not selected against it? There are only two possible reasons for its persistence. Either it must occur beyond the critical stage for natural selection—that is, after the breeding period for the individual has passed, thus becoming irrelevant for evolutionary processes—or there must be something in its very nature, bound up intimately with our biology, which makes cancer recur and recur.

Sometimes it is a valuable exercise to be theoretical, to step away from the suffocation and restraints of excessive data and indulge in fantasy. All the scientists I met were more than happy to do this with me, though they would not have dreamed of publishing their speculations. A book like *An Anthology of Half-Baked Ideas* is a scientific rarity, for in it, scientists were deliberately invited to break out of the constricting bonds of professional caution and wallow, in print no less, in a sea of speculation. But one must remember not to put more weight on speculation than the empirical facts permit. Though the ideas I learned do have a firm foundation in experiments, at this stage they serve as no more than a general guide to theories that may subsequently prove to be of value. The process itself is valuable, however, for it provokes questions, and where questions are provoked, possible answers are stimulated.

Wild speculation can be as dangerous in science as on Wall Street. To indulge out of sheer gambling instinct is foolish. There has to be some likely payoff, and it is as well to have some capital of knowledge and reputation on which to draw. At the height of his fame, a most distinguished scientist, J. B. Bernal, was discussing some very wild scientific ideas with his son, who was also a scientist. His suggestion that they publish a paper together was met by the response, "It's all very well for you, Dad, but I've got my career to consider." The three scientists who were to speculate with me, and show me a few of the most intriguing current ideas, are all at different stages of their scientific careers. They have varying amounts of experience, reputation and daring, so if they are wrong, what they stand to lose varies too.

I went to see the eldest of them, Dr. Aaron Bendich, in his laboratory on the fourth floor of the Sloan-Kettering laboratories in Manhattan. By then I knew a great deal about his solid distinction in cell biology, so much so that I was somewhat subdued. Kingsley Sanders had once telephoned him with one of my incessant questions, prefixing the request with, "Aaron, I know you're a genius," a statement that clearly gave great satisfaction to both parties. He is a small, impish man, in his late fifties, who peered at me very carefully over his spectacles, trying to decide, I am now convinced, whether I was ripe for teasing. I was—and always am. My fear about bothering busy scientists with questions that may appear trivial or ill-considered makes me a natural sucker for any scientific con for at least five minutes. So when Aaron said, "Come over here. I want to show you something," I followed him obediently and in deadly seriousness. He led me to a cheap apparatus which consisted of a spinning drum, with a central upright rod attached to which were two separate glass columns, stranded and twisted to a double helix. "I can separate the two strands of DNA quite easily, you know, by applying a shear force." He pressed a button and the bottom of the machine began to whirl. "There you are," said Aaron. "Drop the DNA molecule in the top, set the machine going and the two strands just split like that." For all of fifteen seconds I believed him; I nearly said, "My God!" but I looked at his face in time. "It works wonderfully with pompous senators and visiting pundits," he said wickedly. I deduce that the machine was built for the purpose of "visitor-testing," so that Aaron can quickly take their measure!

He led me back to his desk and asked, "What do you want to know?" I was still not certain if we were serious now, so I couldn't organize my thoughts quickly enough. He quickly turned the tables again and to my horror asked me a question. "What would happen," he said, "if I mix the sperm of a mouse with the egg of a mouse, given that the egg contained the full complement of chromosomes, instead of the usual half which is normal at fertilization?" I resisted the temptation to say, "I bet you know," for I knew that was precisely what he had been studying recently. As if in apology, he insisted that it was, indeed, a worthwhile question, for the problem of turning the genes on or off may be one aspect of cancer. In cancer, genes are turned on again which earlier in the development of the embryo had been turned off. We know this is so because gene products normally only found in embryos appear in cancer cells. So Aaron said, "Let's invert the question. Suppose the embryonic genes were not being expressed in adult cells, but we found the triggers that could activate these genes in the laboratory, and we pulled them. Would a cell become cancerous?" Up to now, so far as scientists are concerned, the mechanisms for pulling these internal triggers in a cell are capricious and random. What would happen if we could control them externally? What could we do? Could we transform cells? We don't know. In the same vein, he reminded me that 99 percent of all mouse cancer cells have on their surface that telltale antigen, the foetal protein, which is normally only found in their embryos. We know this, yet he asked, "Is the foetal antigen a consequence of cancer or a precondition for it?" I couldn't answer this, nor can anyone, but, Aaron explained, the art of cancer research has at last developed far enough for such precise questions to be asked.

He then showed me a whole series of photographs of cells at various stages and said, "We are going to go on having great difficulty in this field unless and until we can look at a particular cell and say, 'This one is now cancerous and this one is not,' and we can't do this yet." What, then, was the significance of speculation in a field as loose as this? I asked. "But it is important to dream and fantasize," he insisted, "and it is still possible to do this in cancer research without being either spat upon or nailed down. For we are faced with such a crazy series of unknowns, and how can we formulate questions about what is unknown? But we must try. So why not argue now?" he contended. "Formulate what you understand, dissect out the questions, push out from the areas you know, and then see where you go, remembering that beyond lies rigorous experiment. To be too specialized at this stage will do no good." A conjecture need not be loose, however; it can be directed. I reminded Aaron of a device that successful scientists have often used: putting oneself in the situation of the object of study. So a quantum physicist might ask, "Suppose I were an electron, what properties would I need?" "Suppose I were a cancer cell?" I asked. "What would I have to do?"

Clearly, I'd have to make more of myself, he said, and I'd have to find ways of surviving in competition with normal cells. The crucial property could be characterized as total social irresponsibility. The only difference between a cancer cell and a normal cell is that the normal cell responds to pressures, both internal and external. Both cells divide extensively, but when signals

from the outside—from the hormones or the immune system—
indicate that a cancer cell should stop dividing, they are not
noticed, misread or ignored. The cancer cell must therefore have
a system to ward off or circumvent these signals, or could even
have various devious devices for hoodwinking the body into
believing that the signals are being obeyed so the body can now
stop sending them. Suddenly, thousands of miles away from
where I had met them, I was reminded of the Turkomans: each
case of oesophageal cancers began as a single aberrant cell, and
some forty years after that initial event, someone dies. "Why
does it take so long?" I asked Aaron. "I haven't the slightest
idea," he replied, and solemnly took out a file labelled *Questions for Students*, and equally solemnly wrote, "Why does it
take so long?" on the page. Actually he does have some ideas,
though he knows that he can probably garner some more from
his students. "We know there are two stages," he said. "There is
an initiation, the occurrence of a primary event, and then there
is the promotion. If you paint a particular carcinogen on mouse
skin and then later, very much later, paint that skin again with
croton oil you will always get a tumor, *whatever the time*
between the two events. The initial paint leaves a memory at the
site, but the memory requires the application of croton oil to
induce the cancer which was triggered by the first event. During
the promotion the cells divide when ordinarily they wouldn't."
   Most adult cells don't divide frequently, and you don't get
cancer unless a cell *is* in the process of dividing. The trigger
induces a biochemical lesion, but the promotion induces the
frequent divisions. So given an initial lesion—an error in the
cell—there will be a wholesale perpetuation of this error;
ultimately, this is what cancer is, an error in the genetics of
somatic cells. But what triggers it? In a cancer like cancer of the
oesophagus, you are looking at the consequence of an event you
cannot see. In the same way we see the sun as it was eight
minutes ago and not as it is now, in an oesophageal cancer
patient, one sees a consequence of something which happened
years before; looking at it *now* will not tell us what happened
years ago.
   "So there's a lesion you can see. Big deal!" said Aaron. "So
there are viral genes in cancer. Big deal! But what does this really
tell us?" What indeed? Chemicals or viruses or somatic events

all induce breaks in the chromosome which may be perpetuated and which have to be ripened. Is this all we know? Actually we know a great deal more, but I was remembering Aaron's warning, "At this stage to be too erudite, too specialized, will do no good." A fine balance is needed to walk the tightrope between unfettered imagination and a blindered obsession with data, and only the very best scientists achieve, let alone maintain, a successful balance.

It is rare to find someone who is in science because he enjoys total mental freedom—is able to revel in his own imagination. Dr. Jim Trosko is most unusual in this respect. "I wouldn't be in science," he told me, "if I wasn't able to do the 'sloppy' stuff I do. But it pays off in an ability to contribute to the overall picture." In many respects, this made him an ideal person to give me a comprehensive picture of the molecular biology of cancer, and answer my question: Why is cancer still around?

We have been friends for five years now. For a semester each year I go to Michigan State University as a visiting professor, and Jim and I are colleagues in the College of Human Medicine, he as a researcher and teacher. A gentle, bearded man, he looks as if he has stepped out of an Oberammagau Passion Play or at least emerged from another, far less specialized era. He loves to cross intellectual borders, which he does with an ease and facility similar to that of nineteenth-century travellers, who could move from country to country without having to bother about a passport. Jim recognizes no boundaries, though he is aware that other people do. He is clearly astonished that they bother to erect those fences that so hamper communication. He will talk about science and literature, or science and culture, or biology and ethics, or imagination and freedom, all the time setting them in terms of his own unified vision of the world, which he only wishes everyone would see and share. The goal of science— his goal—is unified patterns—not discoveries, not the facts, not therapies, not techniques. Once he has found or sensed the pattern, he is well satisfied. So he does not have that single-minded, obsessional drive for understanding in all its detail— "that fanatical impulse," he calls it. Given the general outline, he is happy to paint in some data, though this will not hold him for long. I have never managed to understand the process or background that gave him this unusual attitude, which is sometimes quite superb and sometimes quite unreal.

Educationally there seems to be no obvious decisive influence. His father was a foundry worker, and Jim maintains that if it hadn't been for *Sputnik* he probably would have been one too. *Sputnik* went up as Jim was in high school; amongst other things, this one engineering feat stimulated a spate of educational programs for young people, with opportunities for careers in science, as part of a long-term bid to keep abreast of the Russians. He became, he says with a rueful grin, "part of America's arsenal against Russia."

He wrote his thesis on radiation genetics, so eventually he went to work in the laboratories of the Atomic Energy Commission at Oak Ridge, Tennessee—the mecca for studies in this area. Acting as liaison between the radiation physicists and the real biologists, he got caught up in the problem of DNA repair, and then drifted into cancer in an entirely serendipitous way. But he did begin to proselytize out there, too, for when he was invited to talk to the staff seminar he spoke about the humanities of science, rather than its content, and how science should have close ties with the worlds of politics, philosophy and history. Some of his colleagues, discomforted by having their intellectual strait jackets ripped off, reacted as if his ideas were the subversive wedge of the counterculture. If this is subversion, it is valuable subversion, even though one eventually becomes sensitized against the edge of rhetoric, however gently spoken.

How does his cosmic vision bear on the science he does? Very little, I would say, when considered in terms of today—small empirical advance, squeezed out from the tightly organized experiment whose conditions are carefully ordained and most rigidly controlled. But away from the bench everything goes, for he would like to construct comprehensive world-pictures and great unifying theories, setting everything into one framework, partly, I believe, as a consoling spiritual comfort against the iniquities of this world. But even within a small area of science once a pattern is found he will be off looking for more patterns in other areas. Indeed, he spoke to me of how his own research interests might now switch away from cancer towards mental health. Of course it is much too premature to switch, or at least it would be for anyone except Jim. For the detailed understanding of cancer in all its ramifications is many years away, but as he now perceives a general theory he must go and look for another one. So the real prizes and successes may well elude him. But it was Jim who brought me to see why cancer is still with us and is likely to remain. The reasons have a beautiful logic.

Though all cells are shielded from outside influences, Jim reminded me, damage to the DNA molecules still occurs. It can come in a variety of ways, with a variety of consequences. If very severe, the damage will be lethal; if not so severe, it may lead to physical defects for an embryo in the uterus. Other influences may induce a genetic change in the cells of the body, and still others will be "carcinogenic"—they will produce a cancerous cell. X-rays can do all four kinds of damage; smoking can induce one or two kinds, and untraviolet light from the sun produces cancer-initiating damage. The damage may cause a DNA chain to break, or one base in the chain may be knocked out or link with something other than another base (a protein, for example), or a whole section of the chromosome may be completely lost. But since the integrity of the DNA must be maintained, whenever there is a break or a lesion, it is repaired.

Consequently, during evolution, mechanisms for repair of DNA have evolved along with the system of DNA molecules itself. By now we know a lot about these mechanisms. Bacteria, yeast, fruit flies, rat-kangaroos and gingko trees—to name but a few species—all have enzymes which repair damage caused by ultraviolet radiation. One must imagine, though not too literally, that there are repair gangs whizzing up and down the DNA ladder. When they spot a lesion, they move in and replace the base, or organize the synthesis of a new section of the DNA molecule and slide it into place like a girder into a bridge. The capacity to do DNA repair is fundamental; its importance can be gauged by the fact that repair mechanisms are found throughout all living systems from the lowest level up. The advantage to the species is clear: repair maintains the integrity of the organism in the face of a whole battery of environmental insults. However, the efficiency of the repair mechanism is itself affected by external influences, and its control is under genetic influence too: if there is repair error in the cells, as long as it isn't lethal, then when the cell divides, that error will be replicated, too.

This leads us straight to the relationship between DNA repair and cancer. There is a genetic disease called xeroderma pigmentosum which is governed by two recessive genes; therefore, a person with it has received the gene that controls it from each of his parents. It shows itself by the most appalling sensitivity to the sun, for such a person exposed to ultraviolet light acquires all types of skin cancer. Most people have enzymes that are capable of repairing ultraviolet lesions, but cultured cells from these patients show that though the lesions are there, the repair systems are quite ineffective. The cells can repair physical damage or damage by X-rays, but not ultraviolet damage. Where the sunlight pours on the skin, lesions are induced, and whereas in a normal person they would be repaired, now they accumulate. If the cells then go into rapid division, a skin cancer finally appears, and the body is quite unable to do anything about it.

Where genetic damage can be totally repaired in the cell, all is well. When it is not repaired at all, there is always a problem. Where it is repaired in a faulty manner, there may or may not be a problem, depending on the level of the existing damage. There seem to be two types of repair: repair free of error and error-prone repair. Jim spoke of the hypothesis that is currently being tossed around: that evolution itself may have *selected for error*. This may have good consequences for the species, though not for the individual.

It comes back to the old argument presented at the beginning of the chapter. We badly need variation, most especially in our germ cells, the eggs and the sperm that are going to give rise to the next generation. When biologists began to speculate about the source of this variation, they looked toward the odd cosmic ray or the swapping of genetic material in the chromosomal dance that the cells go through before the eggs and sperm are finally produced. Or they just called the whole process of variation "mutation." There may be another way of looking at mutation; it may be only a variation that arises from error-prone repair mechanisms, errors overlooked by the cell. If not so gross as to be lethal, these errors are sufficient to provide the necessary variety for the species. All would be fine if this were confined to the reproductive cells alone, but there seems no way of ensuring that it will be. As far as we as individuals are concerned, evolution has slipped up at this point, but when has the evolutionary process ever been concerned with the individual? A minute error in the germ cell just before it is to be fertilized is good for the species. A similar error in repair in an adult skin cell going into a rapidly dividing stage is potentially very dangerous. What the species has not managed to do during evolution is to confine the error-prone mechanisms to the germ cells and the error-free ones to the body. I came to see that the answer to my own initial question, "Why if cancer is so bad, it is not selected out?" is "Because it doesn't matter for the species *one way or another.*" If cancer appears after breeding, as it so often does, it is of no consequence to the race at all. It is just another expression of what Tennyson knew only too well when he wrote about evolution in his great poem *In Memoriam*:

> So careful of the type she seems,
> So careless of the single life.

The only way this could be avoided is if individuals had died of cancer before they bred. Then cancer would have been selected out. But it hasn't happened this way. For cancer comes, on the whole, late in the life cycle.

If all this is true, then what follows? Firstly, that we will *never* eradicate cancer. Both statistics and evolution predict that it is bound to occur in a proportion of individuals, *for it is a price that we as individuals pay for the life of man as a species.* This is the central paradox. It is very deep and intellectually very appealing. Though personally it may be tragic, we must live with it.

Yet there are other paradoxes to come, Jim said. Cancer also links up with aging, another unwelcome property of life. Here we see another link between error, cancer and death, relating to the Hayflick phenomenon, named after the man who first discovered it. If you take a piece of human tissue, such as lung or heart, and culture cells from it, something changes. Oval cells, fibroblasts, appear out of a culture first. A culture of such cells will only survive for between fifty to one hundred divisions of the cells. After about fifty divisions, the time it takes to double the cell population gradually increases; then the whole process stops, and you cannot use the culture any longer. The cells seem to be programmed for a certain time span, a given finite number of divisions—and no more. Paradoxically, the only exception to this rule is when these cells have become malignant; then the converse is true: malignant cells go on forever. The HeLa cells, derived from the woman patient with cervical cancer, form one such line. Though you can't test the extent of their malignancy by pushing them into a human being to see if they get cancer, all the cells of these immortal lines have both an abnormal number of chromosomes and a substantial variety of malignant properties. While normal fibroblast tissues age in tissue culture, those which are malignant do not. Some scientists say this is just a phenomenon of tissue culture, that it bears no relationship to what goes on in organisms and no inferences can be drawn from it. For them this paradox, expressed as "Have cancer and live forever," is a pseudo-paradox. However, for those scientists who take the idea seriously, who believe the phenomenon is genuine and not an artifact, it suggests a relationship between aging and cancer which is not just sheerly coincidental. The fact remains that in tissue culture the only release from aging and death is to become cancerous. But just why remains a matter of speculative theory.

A theory of aging which connects it directly with error, and therefore cancer, originated ten years ago with Leslie Orgel. A cell may on occasion make a wrong protein, but unless the protein is one of those enzymes involved in protein synthesis, this doesn't matter. The cell can always make another protein and discard the fiasco. The rate at which wrong proteins are made is certainly very low, but there is undoubtedly a definite "rate of protein error." If the error involves the mechanism of protein *synthesis*, one mistake results in an accumulation of mistakes in all future synthesis. The error can occur anywhere in the sequence. It is perfectly possible for the genes to be functioning properly and giving out the right message, but if the proteins which put amino acids into position have mistakes in them, the wrong substances are going to be put in. For each error made, ten more errors may result and each of these give ten more. Ultimately you get what Orgel called an "error catastrophe," a molecular *Götterdämmerung*. If there were a genuine link between cancer and aging, then, the argument goes, the longer your life span, the longer you delay having cancer.

The two do seem to be related in some way. Mice get cancer at two years, and they also die of old age at two years. Man gets cancer around seventy and dies of old age around seventy. There are currently two kinds of explanation. The first kind of explanation says that as an animal gets old—whatever old may mean, two years in a mouse or seventy years in a man—things start to go wrong. The things that go wrong make cancer more likely, so that in some sense, *getting old* is a cause of cancer. According to this theory, if we could find a drug which would prevent aging, we would prevent cancer as well. The problem is that we don't really know what causes aging either. It is certainly true that an old person has failing teeth, failing feet, failing lungs, a failing heart and just about failing everything, but we don't know whether these different things happen solely because one time-keeping process, such as the nervous system, has gone wrong, or whether it is because natural selection has just synchronized the machine so that *every part* wears down at about the same time, including repair mechanism cells.

It is likely that the total synchronization of the organism may be all that is at fault. Teeth illustrate this well: an elephant's teeth last as long as an elephant and a mouse's teeth last as long as a mouse. No one can pretend that a mouse's teeth have worn out because there is something in the nervous system that has caused it to happen. Natural selection has simply given a mouse teeth that will last as long as it does. If our built-in repair mechanisms are also similarly programmed for just the same time span, error and therefore cancer are likely to occur at the same time as the other aging processes, and there is no real connection between them.

So those who do postulate a direct connection between cancer and aging, whether because of error catastrophe or the breakdown of the body's defense mechanisms, then have to explain the one gross exception to the general rule: the wide existence of cancer in children. Jim gave me three possible explanations. Firstly, there could be an inherited defect, lesions in cells since birth, that leads to a predisposition for cancer. This could take the form of defective immune systems, or the absence of repair enzymes for cells, or the absence of anti-initiating enzymes (those that render drugs or poisons harmless). Indeed, the reason why some people smoke heavily with impunity and others smoke less and yet get cancer may be due to the absence in the latter group of those enzymes that neutralize the poisons in tobacco. This deficiency is likely to be inherited. Secondly, children with cancer may already have been exposed to environmental hazards. Thirdly, there is a certain degree of probability about cancer. By sheer chance alone, a certain amount of the DNA in cells is always going to mutate, so in any given cell population, some transformed cells are always likely to arise.

These theories—DNA repair, evolution, cancer and aging—may be a little too facile, but they are certainly based on more than the euphoria that comes when two people hold a free-ranging discussion over a glass of wine. On the contrary, Jim himself has contributed to the wealth of solid facts that has been gathered. Though he describes himself as only a "fair to middlin' " scientist, he is too modest. He has already published a bulk of papers on repair mechanisms in mice and hamsters, and grinning with delight, he recently bounded into my office to report another neat, unambiguous result. He induced DNA breaks in Chinese hamster cells with ultraviolent light and then measured the repair at a fine molecular level. Then he repeated the experiment, but added phorbol ester, a constituent of that cancer promoter croton oil. To his delight—and expectation—two things happened. There was such interference with the repair mechanisms that not only was a significant amount of damage repaired with error but the chemical also stimulated the cells to divide fast. So he had produced a classic precancerous condition. At this point he explained, "The excitement was over; the rest is routine. I know what is going to happen." But he had to do the experiment again, with another well-known promoter whose chemical nature and physiological function was very different from the first. As he expected, it had the same effect.

So Jim will continue, with his typical mixture of reflection and experiment, logic and romanticism, science and art. He is doing what he most wants to do. He is aware of the price demanded for real scientific success and states unequivocally that he is not prepared to pay it. He is interested in too many things, so will never stay fiercely and obsessively concentrating on science alone.

. . .

What is the significance of all this audacious theory towards the prevention of cancer or its therapy? Understanding is one thing, practical application another. One must distinguish very sharply between the original event and its consequences, between the first process and the properties that a cell acquires after it has been transformed. First of all, the initial event, however caused, begins with a genetic change. Where we can pinpoint the change and link it to an obvious environmental cause, the problem is easy, for it is one of straightforward avoidance. The cancerous effects of asbestos are undisputed, and people who both smoke and work in asbestos factories are taking a risk comparable to standing up in front of a firing squad and inviting it to shoot. Some remarkable work by Dr. Suzuki and his colleagues at Mount Sinai Hospital, New York, has actually shown that the silicade spicules of asbestos penetrate right into cells. In human cells from cancer patients, these fibers have been seen in the nuclei right amongst the genetic material. The possibility is an intriguing one: somehow the spicules may actually tear at the DNA molecule. They are small enough to do this, and the damage will of course affect the properties of the cell. Here the precautions are very obvious; prevention rather than therapy is the issue.

Secondly, when we know very precisely the consequences of genetic damage, we may be able to do something therapeutically. Dr. Nancy Hogg, working in the laboratories of Avrion Mitchison at University College, London, has developed a neat technique for lifting off molecules from the cell membranes of mice fibroblasts. When cells differentiate normally, they produce a substance which stops them from dividing when they come in contact with other cells. This phenomenon, called "contact inhibition," was initially discovered by Professor Paul Weiss. Now, however, Dr. Hogg has found a massive protein molecule with one of the highest molecular weights known, on the cell membranes of fibroblasts. This may be the recognition molecule, without which the cell does not recognize the others. It is not present on malignant cells, either because it has not been made—the gene for it having been turned off—or because some damage has occurred in the transcription process which prevents the synthesis of the molecule. How we treat the malignant condition will depend on which of these two hypotheses turns out to be true.

These examples touch the effects of malignancy but not the basic cause. I found no difference of opinion whatever on the question of whether or not we will be able to alter or stop a cancerous cell at a genetic level. Not all the scientists I spoke to were as blunt as Sir Macfarlane Burnett, who has said several times, both in public and in print, "So far there has been no human benefit whatever from all that has been learnt from molecular biology." Considered at the level of fundamental genetics, this is true. There is very little that we can yet do or are likely to be able to do concerning a basic change in the internal genetics of the cell. We know a whole battery of genetic disorders: Down's syndrome is Mongolism that results from the abnormality of one chromosome; progeria shows itself as premature aging and comes from an abnormality in a single gene. Its victims are highly likely to develop cancer. Xeroderma pigmentosum and haemophilia are both diseases which result from single gene defects. But what can we do about them, even though we know? Right now, absolutely nothing. Trying to modify the DNA is a skilled and highly problematic job of genetic engineering. With cancer patients, there would be the additional problem of trying to identify a potential cancer cell early in life. That is very difficult, since by the time we know a person has cancer, it is much too late to start looking for the defective initial cell.

But why, one may ask, should we be so pessimistic? Surely it would be possible to change the character of cells by inserting the right gene into the chromosomes, for it has worked most successfully in that old genetic war-horse, the bacterium *E. coli.* However, thirty years of work since the great surge of investigations into phages and bacteria have shaken one of the central dogmas of molecular biology. Once it was said that "what is true in *E. coli* is true in man," but the complexity in man has been shown to be of such a different order that the dogma no longer applies.

For instance, scientists would like to repair genetic deficiencies by delivering some DNA into a defective cell. But you cannot put the DNA in naked, since the enzymes of the cell will chew it up. It would need to be wrapped in a protective protein coat and delivered *via* a virus, in a shield of molecular invisibility. A virus can be incorporated into a bacterium and the viral genes will be expressed. You can deliver a virus into a mouse and the viral DNA is actually incorporated into the nucleus of the animal's cell too. But the viral genes are *never expressed*, for they are suppressed by the host cell. Thus while in theory all is possible, human beings and mice are not the same as bacteria, and we have no reason to suppose that having inserted the gene into the appropriate human cell, it would slide neatly into the nucleus and the whole mechanism would now work properly.

Even if genetic engineering is an unlikely method for cancer prevention or cancer cure, however, a young scientist at Sloan-Kettering gave me an excellent illustration of the very real contributions that molecular biology can make towards cancer diagnosis and therapy. Another central dogma of molecular biology used to be that "information only goes one way." You could pass genetic information from a nucleic acid to a protein, but the information would never go from a protein to a nucleic acid; information would pass from a DNA molecule to a RNA molecule, but not vice-versa. The material of the nucleus was supreme. Biologists were shattered when it was first announced that the dogma did not always hold.

There are, it will be remembered, viruses of two kinds: those with DNA at their genetic core and those with RNA. The RNA viruses, or Rous viruses (named after Dr. Peyton Rous), will transform cells in culture. We know that the genes of the virus are present because the virus can be rescued! Dr. Howard Temin broke the central dogma with a series of beautiful experiments presented with such modesty that the impact was almost nuclear. (The pun is intended.) He has recently received the Lasker Award for this work. It seems that the Rous virus uses its RNA to synthesize its DNA, and that this is then incorporated into the nucleus of the host. Information, transcription, has gone in the reverse direction, and the process is mediated by an enzyme called, not unnaturally, "reverse transcriptase." Howard Temin doesn't like the name—first used in an article in *Nature* by someone else, it carries a number of intellectual ambiguities —but he is stuck with it. After the storms of incredulity, a flood of work resulted. It is a mad, unusual enzyme; as Dr. Etienne de Harven said to me, in a flash of bemused frustration, "It is a crazy enzyme." But some scientists find it delightful.

Dr. Stuart Marcus of the Sloan-Kettering and Mukund Modak are young, in their twenties, amusing, irreverent and brilliant, a slightly wild pair of scientific Siamese twins who in the daytime are, I believe, joined by a seam down the back of their lab coats. Stuart is often unshaven, though on the day the scientific consultants came to visit his chin was very smooth. He may not always be neat and tidy, but his problem is. I heard him give an account of the work on three separate occasions, and I needed those three separate occasions in order to take it in. One such occasion was the informal weekly seminar that Kingsley Sanders called for his group. In a teasing salutation to Temin and the plethora of work on the crazy enzyme, Stuart justified his own problem with an exasperated "There's just got to be something that someone doesn't know about reverse transcriptase!"

It appears that it is quite unlike any other molecule. It is not found in normal white blood corpuscles nor in any normal human tissues. However, Dr. Robert Gallo has done a partial purification and has found the molecule in nearly all patients suffering from acute myeloblastic leukaemia. This is the insidious form of blood cancer that finally executed Stewart Alsop; it is possibly caused by RNA viruses, the ones that make this enzyme. The question that interests Stuart is "Could one use reverse transcriptase as a test for malignancy; more importantly, could one use it as a test for the efficacy of chemotherapy in leukaemia patients?" Certainly it can be used as a test for malignancy, if detected, but so little is produced by the leukaemic cells that it is very difficult to get enough. What Stuart has developed is a sophisticated technique for the isolation of reverse transcriptase in one step. He had an idea, he tried it out, and it worked. He admits that he was very lucky, for techniques rarely work the first time one tries them. Up to now, unfortunately, one needs a tremendous volume of cells in order to detect the enzyme at all. One has to bleed the patient almost dry, put the blood through a kind of "cream separator"—to separate the white blood corpuscles from the red—and go on from there. But Stuart believes his technique, which utilizes a very specific interaction to pick out the molecule he wants, will give a very high yield from a relatively small amount of blood. The particular method, radio-immuno assay, is the most sensitive method for detecting the presence of any protein. If he could obtain a large volume of reverse transcriptase, he would make an antiserum to it and use it to develop an ultrasensitive method to detect the enzyme; if he could do *that*, then he would only have to take a small sample of blood from any patient. If reverse transcriptase was there, even in a minute quantity, it would react with his antiserum; then doctors wouldn't have to drain the patient in order to find out if the enzyme was around.

Why is this important, leaving aside the fact that it is obviously important not to drain the blood of a seriously ill person? The reason has to do with the pressure on a patient. Therapy for leukaemia is very rugged. The therapeutic procedure involves drugs that kill the malignant cells, but the techniques are not yet discriminating enough, so most of the cells in the bone marrow are also killed. Consequently, the patient is prey to all sorts of infection, and the whole therapeutic procedure can be very traumatic both for the doctor and the patient, as I was to see with Rachel. Now, as the incidence of the malignant cells goes down, one would also expect the quantity of reverse transcriptase in the blood to go down too. It begins to decrease at the onset of chemotherapy, and its quantitative measure may prove to be an index of the state of the disease. The moment the malignant cells are killed and the patient goes into remission, you want to halt the chemotherapy; as soon as the disease begins to show itself again, you must start up once more. At the moment, however, there is no accurate technique for marking these stages.

Of course, the significance of this crazy enzyme doesn't stop here. If it is absolutely essential for the growth of tumors caused by RNA viruses, then we could possibly stop the tumor if we could stop the production of reverse transcriptase. If it were also the case that the presence of this enzyme was necessary for the division and replication of metastasizing cells, then again we could stop the spread of cancer by stopping the production of reverse transcriptase. This crazy enzyme is not found in normal cells, and therefore a therapy which acted on it directly would not affect normal cells. At this point the only drugs we know that halt reverse transcriptase production effectively halt many other enzymes too. If we knew the unique properties of the reverse transcriptase molecule exactly, we could match a drug to it.

To do this we will need, for a start, a large number of human leukaemic cells as a source of the enzyme. They are not in plentiful supply. About three kilos of white blood cells can come from one patient at any one time. This may seem a decent enough quantity, but since there is a great deal of research going on into human leukaemia, research laboratories all over the world compete fiercely for these cells. The clinical arm of the center, Memorial Hospital in Manhattan, is of course an important source of material; to get on the list for a "human leukaemic cell appropriation," the project has to go through the Clinical Investigation Committee for approval and allocation. A scientist has to make a case for his priority, stating his problem and experiments very precisely, explaining just what he proposes to do and why, altogether being forced to demonstrate genuine good purpose. It also helps if he can get the head of the haematology department fired with enthusiasm! If two scientists competing for the same supply make equally good cases they may end up by sharing it. A man's seniority and status may give him an edge, but only if these are wedded to a reputation, for these appropriations are taken very seriously indeed. With both youth and inexperience initially working against him, Stuart had, up to that time, very low priority. But after the meeting of the scientific consultants when, with his amusing amalgam of competence, deference and irreverence, he described his work to the board, I got the impression that his rating would change. He had to be exact, however. Bob Good asked him how many cells he needed. I was amused to see that Stuart kept evading the question. Bob persisted and persisted and finally said flatly, in a manner that could not be ignored, "How much do you need?" Stuart positively gulped, then disgorged the amount. "A kilo," he finally replied. His reluctance came not because of uncertainty about either his methods or his sums, but because he knew that he was asking for an awful lot. Four months later, his project was approved, subject to his establishment of protection for the work. Human cancer cells are potentially hazardous material and are not just thrown around.

I had a great time talking to Stuart and Mukund. They are very different from Jim, for they both have that obsessional drive for exact detailed knowledge. The creative imagination is there, all right, but once a problem is defined they will work it out all the way, ferreting out the last minute piece of information, leaving no theoretical loopholes at all if they can help it. The combination of concern, superb competence and downright irreverence as they practice science is a wonderful mixture, one which prevented me from taking myself too seriously. Cheerfulness always kept breaking in. Stuart was quite unconsciously revealing. Someone mentioned the elegance of his experiments, to be countered with, "Oh, an elegant experiment is only one that no one else has done." Asked how long it would take him to get the Nobel Prize, he returned the compliment with his neat reply: "About five years after you do."

He is in cancer research not just to take intellectual ego trips, but because he has a long-felt personal concern. His family has been riddled with cancer. His father died of it, and his grandmothers, too, on both sides. He told me he would have liked to have been a medical doctor but would be far too emotionally involved. He discovered at an early age that he wouldn't be able to stand telling somebody that they might die. "I might not be able to cure a patient, but at least I can help," he said. He is so obviously incapable of prevarication that the politics of scientific research, shown by occasional infighting and clashes have already disillusioned him, could in the end defeat him. I think it unlikely, though, for most scientists have to suffer through this. He will survive because his deep motivation will carry him through. Battered at times, but still thoroughly in love with science, he will surge ahead, determined never again to be pushed around but just to keep on practicing scientific research. "After all," he says, "someone has to keep doing that." The rest of us can be thankful that someone is.

In those heady, golden days when molecular biology was young and most molecular biologists were too, Jacques Monod described a typical laboratory. It contained, he said, a number of bright young men in polo-necked sweaters and glasses, who would argue for two weeks in an atmosphere of fevered excitement as they discussed a particular experiment, only to decide in the end that it was not worth doing. That was twenty-one years ago, and the subject has come of age. A general theory of cancer, if it comes, will be firmly embedded in the matrix of the two great unifying theories of biology: evolution and molecular biology. By itself it will give great intellectual satisfaction, but nothing more. But the new generation of young men, facing in cancer an intellectual challenge just as great, are not content to be just theoretical. They are pressing equally hard on the practical applications of the theory, and it is this that will help defeat the disease.

4

CANCER AND IMMUNITY:

IT'S ONLY A TRIAL IF I RECOGNIZE IT

It stimulated the phagocytes; and the phagocytes did the rest.

—Sir Ralph Bloomfield Bonington
(*The Doctor's Dilemma,*
George Bernard Shaw)

TUMORS HAVE BEEN KNOWN to go away of their own accord. It doesn't happen very often, but when it does the effects are dramatic. Until recently there has been a vacuum of explanation into which saints and quacks have stepped, invoking faith, wonder drugs, diets, regimes. Their explanations do not stand up under examination, but the fact of spontaneous remission is genuine. Doctors are used to unexpected results, and the unexpected sometimes happens without anyone doing anything. For some considerable time, the existence of spontaneous remissions provided the strongest single piece of evidence for those scientists who were betting on immunology as an effective way to attack cancer. These incidences might have been rare, but they provided encouraging evidence even as late as six or seven years ago, for while there was good reason to believe that there was an immune reaction to tumors in laboratory animals, there was virtually no evidence whatever that there was an immune reaction in man. Consequently, those scientists who were prepared to back the immunological horse invested a great deal in the fact of spontaneous regression and also to immunological reaction as its explanation. But scientists no longer need this piece of evidence, for new techniques for measuring these reactions show that there is, in all cases, an immunological response to a tumor on the part of a patient.

Scientific confidence in cancer immunology no longer needs to be boosted. It is a discipline which is doing a roaring trade, enjoying a period of intellectual prosperity unanticipated ten years ago. Under the effervescent direction of Robert Good, the atmosphere around the immunological sections of the Sloan-Kettering Institute has something of the quality of a boom town, not so much because of the financial rewards, but because of the promise of great therapeutic payoff. The analogy must be changed, for only one word can describe their activity—volcanic. The subject is fizzing, being carried along by confident whiz kids who periodically erupt in bursts of optimism and data.

The present director of the Sloan-Kettering Institute is one of the most colorful and exuberant figures in the field, who obviously and unashamedly delights in riding the crest of the scientific wave. His energy and enthusiasm are sometimes so overpowering that many other things besides the phagocytes are stimulated when he is around, and most people generally end up being either for or against him. Not only is he unperturbed but he even feels very positive about the reactions of some of the members of the institute who thoroughly disliked what he did in his first months there. Creative conflict, the life blood of both science and political institutions, is clearly essential to him. The tall, robust figure in sneakers, turtleneck and lab coat is likely to remain right in the center of activity, and of controversy as well.

He is now a very busy man indeed, and five o'clock in the morning has been known to be offered as an appointment time. It it is not an hour when most of us are at our intellectual best, but at that time, he is scintillating and poised on the edge of the day's scientific race. I was lucky to get a date at six one evening, and we talked for five hours. There was one enchanting moment as Bob described a time when, as a very young man, he spoke with Karl Landsteiner, one of the greatest names in immunology, and Linus Pauling. They were discussing the properties of the chemicals in the immunological system, trying to relate the structure of the molecules to the fantastic powers of the immune system. Landsteiner turned to Pauling, who even then had a tremendous reputation as a chemist, and said, "What kind of molecule, that we can imagine, would be like that—that could do all these things?" Pauling stretched his hands over his head and said, "Why, a molecule like me." Bob stretched his arms up, too. The shape of the critical molecule is a Y, and this tall, lanky man with his arms held over his head gave a human personification of the immunoglobin molecule.

Understanding the structural and functional Y will help us to answer the why of cancer. Modern molecular biology is expressed in terms of words, information and codes, so perhaps it is not surprising that Bob Good uses linguistic symbols a great deal. He speaks of the "cell's language" which we have to understand. Nobody would worry very much about cancer if it didn't kill you. Since it does, we must make the cells behave, and *tell* them when to stop dividing. In order to do this, we must understand the language of the cell in fine detail, as expressed in the patterns of molecules at the cell surface. For by these molecules the cells communicate to one another and therefore to the body as a whole. We are just beginning to make out the "words." Dr. Ted Boyse, for instance, can induce the development of the T lymphocytes, a critical cell in the immune system, and in a matter of several hours see displayed on the surface of the cells the products of eleven different genes. That is, for each gene he can identify and pull off the cell surface the very protein that the gene is specifying.

Susceptibility to disease can be defined, too, in genetic terms. Chromosomes are now mapped out rather like the routes on cross-country maps given to motorists by automobile associations. Here is a town; there are crossroads. Here on this chromosome is a Locus, No. 4; here, at this point, is a variation in the gene structure, Allele W27. Many family studies of cancer patients are underway to determine the role of genetic influence in malignancy. Eventually, this approach will provide a link to Janez Kmet's work. For instance, all patients with a rapidly progressing form of multiple sclerosis have been found to have a particular genetic structure at one specific locus on the chromosome. But what is it that scientists can manipulate and what can this work possibly do for us? What they are doing, Bob Good emphasized—they all emphasized—is cellular engineering, not genetic engineering. They are not going to affect the basic genetic mechanism at the heart of our clinical problems, and we may never be able to. If cancer arises from a genetic deficiency or aberrancy, all that can be said at that point is "So be it." If people have a predisposition to fast-developing multiple sclerosis because of a certain genetic structure at one particular locus on a chromosome, we may have to take that situation as given, recognizing that it will be very difficult to change. We *can* understand the molecular consequences of such genetics, however, and manipulate or alter the surface proteins in such a way as to influence the behavior of the cell.

The general theoretical outline of immunology is easy to grasp. Nature is always on the alert: the cells of the immune system are constantly prowling about the body like trigger-happy soldiers. The recognition of "foreigners" comes from the clues they leave—the fingerprints that every substance, strange cell or virus carries. The fingerprint is their "antigen," and these can be a variety of chemical molecules. Once the antigens are recognized, the immune cells produce the antidote, the "antibody," a protein which can bind with and thus neutralize the antigen. The test for the existence of the one is its capacity to link with the other, so if Magda's antigen is really the Hodgkin's disease antigen, then it will bind with the corresponding Hodgkin's antibody and no other. The specificity is almost total.

The crucial cells are lymphocytes, part of our white blood cell population, and the crucial organ is a small gland in the chest, the thymus. Two parallel systems are involved in the internal surveillance of the body, and two sorts of lymphocytes are produced. Both come from our bone marrow, but one type, the T cell, has to go to the thymus gland to mature. The other, the B cell, matures somewhere unknown and then goes into the blood system. Their different structures indicate different functions, though the cells will cooperate at times. The T cells deal with the big problems, those that arise in skin grafts, transplants and cancer. The B cells tackle the smaller fry of bacteria, viruses and all infections in the bloodstream.

One property is absolutely indispensable for a system of this kind—a capacity to distinguish those natural cells and substances that belong to the body from those that do not. The system has evolved its own fail-safe mechanism, with the capacity to discriminate "self" from "non-self," so that the body's defense system attacks only the invaders. Actually the mechanism does sometimes fail. The lymphocytes can get diseases too; they can have their own form of cancer, and their capacity for discrimination can become lost, so that they turn upon the body itself. Then we get an auto-immune disease, a personal and biological tragedy. Bob Good has suggested that cancer in the form of auto-immune disease may be a price we pay for this valuable function of "self-recognition." As we saw in the case of viruses, the body responds well to a massive attack, but it has not evolved the capacity to deal with small, sustained, growing sources of antigenic stimulus. One can see why not: if the immune system were to challenge every cellular variation, every small but not serious change, the end result would be literally self-defeating. A cancer, too, begins small. A tumor goes through a period of sustained growth, and this may show the very same pattern of small but gradually increasing antigenicity that the body does not handle so effectively.

Immunology has, from the very beginning, touched medicine and theoretical biology at almost every point. Its history and early development was closely linked with the theory of infectious diseases, so for a long time the answer to the question "Why have we evolved such a system?" was given in terms of protecting the body from lethal bacteria and viruses. During the first thirty years of this century immunology was, according to Sir Peter Medawar, an amalgam of "bare-faced empiricisms and embarrassingly silly terminology, a matter of vaccine and anti-sera and skin tests, and not much else." During World War II, however, there was a sudden burst of activity: in coping with the problem of providing skin transplants for severe burn cases biologists and surgeons had to face the facts of tissue rejection; and this induced a reassessment of the field at a very fundamental theoretical level. Why was it that one's own skin, or that of a close relative, could be made to "take," whereas foreign skin would be sloughed off in a matter of two to three weeks? The evolutionary question is also an intriguing one. Nowhere in the evolutionary history of our species or of any other species could we have encountered or been prepared for transplants. So if animals have such a fantastic capacity for the rejection and destruction of foreign material, its origin must be sought elsewhere. Twenty-five years later, we have another possible answer: the tip of the iceberg theory. This says that those cancers which are actually manifested represent only a small proportion of those we have or have had, and that the biological purpose of the immune system—its evolutionary raison d'être—is to recognize and deal with the aberrant cells. But sometimes a few slip through the defensive network, or the ecology of the surrounding cells selects one transformed cell and it is "permitted" to grow.

This is an attractive unifying theory which makes a great deal of sense. In addition, it is extremely challenging both for the scientist and the clinician . . . if it is true. But such is the youth of this field that this year I heard the theory being firmly denied by a scientist who had equally fervently espoused it only a few years back. This was not inconsistency but a reflection of the state of the art. The evidence is not yet watertight. As Bob Good insisted, immunology in relation to cancer is still largely an empirical art. The connections are there, but their nature is far from clear. Before I started this work I talked with Sir Peter Medawar, and my final question was, "Have you any general warnings to give me as I go into this?" He certainly had, for he said, "Don't forget that the weight of opinion in cancer research shifts as rapidly and unpredictably as unsecured ballast in a merchant vessel in the Bay of Biscay. Don't be too confident about anything." It was a good warning.

But the air of a gold-rush town is heady wine indeed, and there is no mistaking the mood. This doesn't mean that the whole of cancer is going to buckle under a frontal attack from immunologists, but it is an area ripe for exploiting. It is easy to be swept away on the tides of euphoria and conviction, so when assessing the present achievements and future promise of the work I had to keep my head. I asked half a dozen separate people in New York, where I should turn for a cool appraisal, who should be my devil's advocate. They all said, "Go to England. See Peter Alexander and Avrion (Av) Mitchison."

So with my critical antennae quivering, I went to University College, London, a very different place from the Sloan-Kettering

Institute. If Sloan-Kettering has qualities of a gold-rush town, then University College has the air of those sedate cathedral-cities in the novels of Anthony Trollope. History stalks the shadows; the traditions are secure, the atmosphere gently complacent, even a little smug at times, and the ghosts literally linger in its corridors. Whenever I go down the main hall I feel that I should pull my forelock to the embalmed corpse of Jeremy Bentham, one of the founders of University College, sitting in frozen silence in his glass-fronted box, preserved for eternity and meetings of the council. It is a great way to get a quorum. But in the Department of Zoology the ghosts are more alive and immediate; one doesn't have to be dead to provide a haunting spirit. So Avrion's immediate predecessor, John Maynard Smith, rubs shoulders with Sir Peter Medawar. And through the late D. M. S. Watson, a comparative anatomist, we go back to Ray Lankester, the professor at the turn of the century. Here in these spirits, the evolution of biology is captured, for in intellectual preoccupations and available scientific tools, Lankester and Watson with their classical interests were far closer together than Watson with his bones is to Avrion with his lymphocytes. Intellectual light-years separate these two men, and one gets a curious feeling walking down the dark, narrow corridors. If one night Avrion in his clogs met Ray Lankester in his ghostly chains, on what common zoological ground could they possibly meet? For Avrion is a product of a different era. Molecular biology may not encompass the whole of biology, but it transformed it, bringing a totally new dimension to the science.

Considered in intellectual terms, Avrion Mitchison comes from a very distinguished pedigree indeed, heir to an academic tradition which still preserves something of its old ambience. The beautiful brass microscope which sits on the window ledge in his room may even have been handed down from professor to professor, a symbol of scientific apostolic succession. But his personal pedigree is equally notable. His two brothers are brilliant scientists too, and J. B. S. Haldane was his uncle: a superb biologist, Haldane gave a most moving account of his own cancer shortly before he died. Avrion spent much of his childhood in a vast rambling house in the Scottish Highlands, a kind of intellectual Hyannis Port, bathed in a constant stream of

mental stimulus and cold water. Behind this family the ties
stretch back into the nineteenth century, bound to those of the
Huxleys, the Darwins and the Wedgwoods. Much of the great
intellectual flowering in nineteenth-century England was in
science both pure and applied, and families like these are
consciously aware of this tradition and utterly assured in the
background it gives them. Intellectual brilliance and wide
knowledge are taken for granted. At the worst this self-assurance
can be manifested as an intolerable arrogance; at best, as in
Avrion, it is matched to a deceptive air of relaxed effortlessness.
The assumption is always made: everyone is equally clever and
equally widely read. So the talk proceeds in a series of quantum
jumps, as Avrion moves five steps ahead in each argument,
confident that the steps in between are obvious—which they are
to him.

On the one hand, he is the most unlikely person to cast in the
role of devil's advocate, those acid-minded, reactionary cardinals
in the Vatican's Curia. Avrion is neither acid-minded nor
reactionary. But on the other hand, with his obvious qualities of
competence and solidarity, he is a natural for the role. Nothing
is going to slip past him. If immunologists fielded a soccer team
for the Scientific World Cup, he would be the goalkeeper.
Opponents' shots are stopped kindly, not aggressively, but with
such firmness as to be maddeningly frustrating.

The society from which Avrion emerged cheerfully tolerated,
even welcomed, the amiable eccentric. The carpet slippers that
as a student he made a point of always wearing in the laboratory,
have been replaced by large wooden clogs whose "clomp,"
"clomp," "clomp" down the corridor is a familiar sound. This,
and his permanent—or so it seems—Shetland sweater, denote a
creature of habit, and add up to that air of absent-minded
unworldliness which Bertrand Russell missed so much in the
American academic. It is all terribly deceptive, however: it hides
a real toughness of body and mind that runs through the family.
Physical fitness was almost a fetish for Uncle J.B.S., and even
this had its benefits for science. He would experiment on himself
and once wrote a fascinating paper, "On Being One's Own
Rabbit." He chose to do this not for reasons of moral
excellence, but because his body would provide such a superb
subject. Avrion would do this too. Add to all this the assured

background, and the result is a scientist who has advanced, firmly and deliberately, onto a piece of intellectual territory, planted his flag, declared it his own, and knows *every* square inch in great detail.

Avrion came into immunology in the most ordinary way, he told me. He first took a degree in biology, but when it came to doing a thesis, he wasn't at all certain which way to go. He was captured, he says, by personalities rather than by scientific promise, and after meeting Sir Peter Medawar at Oxford, signed on with him. Ten years later, after interludes in America and Edinburgh, he returned to work with Sir Peter at the Medical Research Council in Mill Hill, London, doing basic immunology. Three years ago he began to concentrate his effort on tumor immunology. He was one of the few scientists I talked to who came right out and admitted that he had been wrong about something. Twelve years ago, he was in America to give a paper at the inauguration of a new research laboratory in California, a cancer center that was going to have an "immunological angle to it." He remembers being extremely sceptical about cancer immunology in his paper, and this scepticism had a great deal to do with the history of the subject.

Tumor immunology got off to a very unfortunate start. Over seventy years ago, Jensen, a Danish pathologist, transplanted tumors from one mouse to another and found that generally after a short growth period the tumor would regress. This seemed proof that tumors could be made to disappear, and that the animal could be "cured." A flood of varied work poured out aimed at understanding and exploiting this fact. Yet when sufficient quantities of highly inbred mice became available in the 1930's, mice which would happily accept tumors from each other, the whole research was totally eroded. Though the scientists had believed that they were studying tumor *regression*, they had actually been studying foreign transplant *rejection*, and at that time there was no way that they could have distinguished between the two. Looking back now, with our years of experience in tissue and organ transplantation, we see that the rejections were nearly always rejections of the transplants. To establish this involved a long uphill fight, what Avrion characterized as "a great deal of scientific fuss and bother." Once it was clear, however, transplants supplanted tumors as the focus of people's interests and thoughts. Things stayed like this for a while, for fashion operates in science just as much as in design. Consequently, twelve years ago, when Avrion gave his paper, there was a great deal of excitement, but not about tumor immunology. The transplant antigens had been just discovered and analyzed, and a "very beautiful picture" was emerging. All the talk about antigens specific for tumors seemed not only to be confusing the issue, but to be quite mistaken, and Avrion thought so too.

Yet history continued to provide curious twists and coincidences. It now appears that tumor regression and transplant rejection may be very closely linked after all. We know that in the early stages of the tumor the host actually *is* reacting vigorously, yet the tumor avoids destruction. In the early stages of a skin graft or a heart transplant, the host reacts equally vigorously, in the same way and through the same system, yet in that situation the graft is destroyed. So one can ask a very precise question. What is it that allows a tumor to slip through the net of immunological security in the face of an active immune response, the very same response which guarantees that a transplanted heart will be destroyed? Here is another paradox: avoiding destruction constitutes a failure for cancer therapy, but a success for the transplant surgeon. Consequently cancer therapists and transplant surgeons are now asking the same question: How do tissues avoid destruction? One can turn this question around: Are there any circumstances in which aberrant tissues in the body are clearly *not* rejected? Cancer seems to be one example; pregnancy is another. The foetus produces antigens which are recognized as "foreign" by the mother, but still the embryo is not expelled. The question then becomes even more precise: Is there a molecular structure which functions chemically to prevent recognition of foreigners? How do both a foetus and a cancer hoodwink the system? The answer seems to be: in precisely the same way!

Sometimes as one looks at an area of science, the problems seem too unwieldy, the issues too complex, the facts too disparate, the contradictions too baffling. This is how it has been with cancer immunology. A scientist must hang in there, and he can do so because he knows, in a way which comes from both intuition and experience, that the links are there. Somewhere there is a clue and when this is found, a great deal will begin to fall into place. We are just at one such point, and the realization comes as a wondrous relief. Cancer has an Achilles heel: to avoid destruction, a tumor may be using the very same mechanism that a foetus does. It is clear that many of the antigens produced by malignant cells are very similar to those produced by embryos. The process of malignant transformation reawakens antigens from the embryonic stages. Now that we know, it is perhaps not too surprising, for both situations are periods of active cell division. In the early embryonic stages there is a tremendous spurt of cell division; there is another in cancer; there is yet a third in psoriasis, a disease in which the skin is scaly and reddened, and the cell metabolism turns over four times faster than normal. The incidence of cancer in people with psoriasis is very low. If cancer and transplants and embryos have something in common—namely, the production of a molecule or molecules generally called the foetal antigens—then it would clearly pay us to find out their character and the nature of their activating trigger. Once we have the chemical characteristics of the antigens, then we can begin to manipulate them. If the presence of a molecule (or molecules) stops the body from recognizing the material as foreign, then in theory we can extract it. By injecting it into patients who have received organ transplants, we could hoodwink the system. In theory, too, we could change the molecular structure of these antigens in cancer patients so that their properties would be altered and they could no longer practice their deceptive role. We could use their existence as diagnostic tests to catch tumors at very early stages.

So three years ago Avrion had solid reasons for switching his attention to the problems of tumor immunology. First of all, he fidgets about the problem of immunological control, and tumor immunology, once it had been established as a genuine fact, gave him the justification for looking at control mechanisms in great detail. He is convinced that the *control* of immunological response is the key to all immunology. Cancers grow in the first place because some control mechanism or other limits the host's immune response, perhaps blocking it and thus allowing the tumor to evade the surveillance mechanisms.

The sheer challenge of the situation was another stimulus for him, for the body's responses to a tumor are comparatively so weak that scientists must think of really clever things to do in order to get anywhere at all. After the control of transplant rejection, a studying of these "blocking factors" promises to provide the next major therapeutic application of immunology. Technologically, too, it was the right time to begin trying, as techniques had finally been developed for analyzing immune reactions between cells in vitro as well as in vivo. Once a problem can be tackled in a culture dish, then it is easier to manipulate since the conditions of an experiment can be changed and controlled. Finally, Avrion emphasized, another important factor in his switch to tumor immunology was the sheer encouragement that everyone received from the genuine success of one or two clinical trials in cancer immunology. With his well-refined sense of intellectual territoriality, Avrion staked out this new claim.

Of all the scientists working on cancer, immunologists gave me the strongest impression, not so much of success as of being able to focus very precisely on a series of intellectual and therapeutic targets. Here I finally sensed, for the first time, just where T. H. Huxley's physician, the "blind man hitting out with a club," will metamorphose into the sniper picking off intruders with lethal accuracy. Speaking with Avrion, one sees how the general problem is dissected into a series of fine elements. The Achilles heel, the foetal antigens, are a most reasonable target, but he has very strong views about these weak antigens. To talk about them in such a general term as a "foetal antigen" merely shows how little we know about them. One might as well talk about an "adult antigen." There are millions of adult antigens, and there are likely to be millions of foetal antigens too. Chop up some embryos, inoculate adult animals with them, and you will get a battery of new antibodies in the blood, indicating that a whole variety of foreign proteins came from your embryos. How many of these antigens are there? What cells do they occur on? What are they doing in foetuses anyway?

Avrion's own particular interests focus on two problems. Firstly, the "blocking factors," the antigens or complexes of antigens and antibodies that somehow block the action of the T. lymphocytes. They have only recently become accessible to study and, as befits an ex-pupil of Peter Medawar's, his interest in them reflects a problem which finally seems soluble. Blocking factors have been known for a long time, but up till now, their reactions and the systems that involve them have been too weak to have been of much use. Many of the reactions of the T. lymphocytes are so strong in vitro, however, that for the first time one can analyze the blocking factors properly, finding out about their size, their chemistry, and just how they interact with the surface of the lymphocytes. The more one can do in vitro, the clearer it all gets, and the very best experiments combine laboratory manipulation of the immune response and compare it with what goes on in the body.

Yet there is still an enormous gap, he cautioned me. The experiments mostly go on in small Petrie dishes, or even in mini-Petrie dishes, which mostly hold less than 1 c.c. of liquid, or they take place in tissue-culture chambers in which all the different cells, fibroblasts and tumor cells are all confronted with lymphocytes. The cells are mixed up with one another, and for some reason the tumor cells are killed. This is a long way from the patient, and this is another problem, which some of Avrion's colleagues are tackling.

Nine months after this research started, the pattern was taking the form of a Tibetan prayer wheel, with the same people, the same ideas and the same problems coming round again. Kingsley Sanders was Avrion's tutor at Oxford for a while. Moreover, Avrion's colleague, Reg Gorczynski, whom I met next, had Bob Williams as his tutor, whose other pupils were also to cross my path (see Chapter 5). Reg Gorczynski is as English as Avrion, in spite of his unpronounceable name. Twenty-six years old, he is the son of a Polish sailor and an English mother. He read chemistry at Oxford and hated it, so in his third year he switched to biochemistry, doing the equivalent of two years' biochemistry in one summer. Reg's ambition is to unblock the blocking factors in cancer. I came to describe his problem as "The Case of the Uncooperative Lymphocytes." He is tackling the problem simultaneously in tissue culture and in mice, doing the same tests in both, so that he can correlate the phenomena in the one with the phenomena in the other. His aim is not only to get a model system for spontaneous regression of tumors, but also to find ways to induce regression. The tumor in the mice is caused by an RNA virus, the Moloney sarcoma virus, and is a tumor which has a rather peculiar relationship with its host. If the tumor is transplanted into a mouse, it grows well, but after a period of time it *always* regresses of its own accord. However, if you take a mouse with this transplanted tumor and irradiate it with a large but not lethal dose, the tumor will grow and grow and never disappear at all. While the tumor is growing and regressing in the control animals, Reg monitors the lymphocytes, taking them out and by tests in vitro asking the questions "What are they doing at this stage? Do they kill the tumor?"

The question "Do they kill the tumor?" is very general when put in that form. Turned into a practical experiment with observations, it dissolves into three more questions, which lead to three different kinds of tests. First, do these lymphocytes in culture react to the tumor antigens in the accepted manner (i.e., you are an antigen, I'll make an antibody against you)? Second, do they, in culture, actually kill off the tumor cells? Third, if you inject them into one of the irradiated mice, do they now protect the animal? Since these mice are now well on the way to dying of their tumors, this is an important question, for the effect of the radiation has been to nullify the attempt of the mouse to kill off the tumor itself. If the mouse is protected from the tumor it can only be because of the lymphocytes.

The answers are becoming as precise now as the questions. All three tests show that the T lymphocytes are the active cells, and that they *are* killing the tumors. But in all three tests, a small proportion of the lymphocytes, some of the B cells, do not cooperate. They block the activity of the T cells. This happens because the tumors have produced yet another antigen which, reacting with the surface of the B lymphocytes, has changed their nature in some way, possibly altering the surface proteins. Fortunately, not every B lymphocyte is affected. The T and B lymphocytes come in a number of subclasses, which luckily can be separated by physical size alone. Each subclass has different functions, too, and it is the B lymphocytes of a certain size which are the crucial ones. If the same situation applies to human beings, we could devise a rational therapy by getting rid of all B lymphocytes of a given size and shape.

This could be done: While in Canada, Reg learned a great deal about techniques of separating cells, using physical characteristics to sort them out in the same way that apples or eggs are graded in a factory. In immunology one tries to understand biochemical properties. Any technique which depends on biochemistry to separate cells may by its very nature alter the very property you are trying to study. However, with physical means there is no problem: You could transfuse the blood of the patient, filter out the cells of the critical size—the "uncooperative lymphocytes"—and put the blood back in. The snag is, of course, that those particular B lymphocytes probably have another, equally important, job to do in the body, for obviously their appearance on our evolutionary stage cannot be only because it proved necessary to stymie the effect of *good* T lymphocytes. They *must* have another function.

Reg's own future is a little uncertain. Like most of the work in this department, his is supported by the Imperial Cancer Research Fund, so his very existence at University College depends upon the continuation of grants. He wants to stay, but financially he wonders whether he can afford to. London is as expensive as New York. Mortgages, down payments and transportation take a big slice of the monthly paycheck of young people, and English postdoctoral fellows are paid on quite a different salary scale than their American counterparts. But he wants to stay if he can, for a very simple reason. "It is quite likely," he said, "that there are places where there are good groups of infinitely clever people to work with, but so far as I am concerned, this is the very best place. I am not good enough to work by myself, and these people are simply the best people I have ever met in science and have ever worked with."

His work is a characteristic example of the basic immunology at the heart of Avrion Mitchison's department. Exciting rather than glamorous or flamboyant, the research neither attracts the headlines nor is it intended to do so. But it is absolutely fundamental, and all the time one edges nearer and nearer to the patient. Here again I met that particular brand of clinician-researcher who moves with ease between the patient and the laboratory. Peter Beverley is another of Avrion's colleagues and also an Imperial Cancer Research Fellow. He qualified as a physician at University College in 1967, did his residency there and for two years worked in general practice in the East End of London. He finally left general practice because he felt he would never be able to satisfy the "touching faith" that patients have in a doctor's capacity and capabilities. Even before he qualified, he had worked one summer with Avrion and Peter Medawar at the Mill Hill laboratories of the Medical Research Council. With this background, it was not surprising that when he was finally established as a full-time research scientist, his interest continued to center around people. What he really wanted to study was not animal tumors and animal immunology, but human tumors and immunology. He needed a variety of experience, so he went to the Sloan-Kettering Institute to work with Lloyd Old and Ted Boyse and finally Robert Good. One gets the impression that he wasn't sorry to come back to London. He returned with very strong feelings about big science as it is practiced in America, and equally strong convictions about the worth and solidity of the work being done in London. There is an entirely understandable defensiveness when he speaks about this. The Sloan-Kettering Institute does, after all, have cash, energy and terrific prestige in cancer research, and he did leave it for a place which in absolute terms is somewhat poorer. But I suspect that he found American science stimulating but far too brash—and besides, he didn't get the research experience with human tumors that he really needed.

Peter Beverley gave me a new detail on the value of immunological studies in cancer as diagnostic tests. In pressing on the problem of cancer, one wants to be doing something useful at once, as well as doing the basic work which will provide the foundations for future therapy. Peter hopes to combine these two aspects by exploiting the property of a tumor to leave its fingerprint, using its antigen both as a diagnostic index to tell us what is happening, and as a prognostic one to tell us what is likely to happen. He emphasized, however, that this is really a short-range problem, with short-range results; that he is simply making a small advance in one direction.

Basically, what he would like to do is take human tumors, and by injecting them or transplanting them into animals, make an anti-serum. From the blood of these animals he would make a fluid containing antibodies that would react to antigens from the same kind of tumor *from human beings*. Thus if you have a patient whom you suspect of having this tumor, a quick blood test should tell you if you are right. You challenge the patient's blood with the anti-serum to the tumor, and if there is an immunological reaction, the point is made. But making the serum is rather complicated, for the "recipe" has to go through several stages.

In cooperation with the surgeons of University College Hospital, he is working on carcinoma of the ovary. He is not yet absolutely confident that he has got an anti-serum that is unequivocally specific for human ovarian cancer, and with native caution he insisted that he would not proceed any further until he was quite certain of this first stage. If and when he is satisfied, however, he will go on and try to pull the telltale antigen out of the tumor and find the molecule that is *the* crucial fingerprint for human ovarian carcinoma. Then he will develop a technique which will enable him to detect it in the very minutest quantity, making a "super anti-serum" that can be used to test a patient's blood for the detection of the carcinoma. There might also be another payoff, for if one could purify this molecule, it might be possible to immunize patients against these tumors. You could give the patient a large shot of the tumor antigen and give the body the kind of massive immunological shock which Bob Good insists it is superbly able to manage. Shaking up the immune system of the patient with "one hell of a jolt" may be the best way to mobilize the defense mechanism. No doubt Sir Ralph Bloomfield Bonington would have predicted this: "It stimulated the phagocytes; and the phagocytes did the rest."

Many moves in current immunotherapy do in fact rely on stimulating the phagocytes in one way or another. These techniques were described by Harold Schmeck of *The New York Times*, in a felicitous phrase, as "a sort of biochemical judo," the art being to exploit the other man's strength in order to defeat himself. One way to make the lymphocytes nervous, to make them recognize changes in cell surfaces and unusual antigens, would be to use nonspecific stimulators. A tuberculosis vaccine, B.C.G., is one such stimulant; George Mathé of Paris, among others, has been using it extensively with patients with advanced leukaemia. But, alas, there are a number of curious difficulties, and the usual number of paradoxes.

In some cases it is clear that not all antibodies are efficient in killing a cancer cell. Worse, it is equally possible that the B. lymphocytes may in fact actually favor the spread of the cancer

by a phenomenon which is called "the enhancement factor."
The explanation is horribly simple: the capacity of a lymphocyte
to attack a cancer cell depends on its recognizing that the tumor
cells are foreign. But if the tumor has been caused by a viral
infection, the B lymphocyte antibody will be produced to
combat the viral antigens, and will, as it were, smear the tumor
with antibodies against the virus. Therefore, the tumor signal
cannot get through, so the T lymphocytes cannot possibly
recognize the tumor. Immunological enhancement used to be
dismissed as an aberrant laboratory puzzle, but unfortunately it
is a very genuine effect. In transplant situations it occurs
again—equally genuine, but this time thoroughly fortunate. If
the foreign graft can be "smeared" and thus shielded from the
effect of the T lymphocytes, then the transplant will take. So
once more there is a Janus-faced quality about immunology, the
two sides of the same coin being tumor evasion and graft
rejection. The only way to solve these linked problems lies in a
thorough understanding of immunology.

One problem in cancer has always been the most insidious,
and here immunology may really come into its own. Very few
people die from the primary tumor. It is the secondary growths,
the metastasizing cells, that are the real criminals, and of all
therapeutic areas, immunology seems likely to be most useful
here. Most tumors of the solid type, however, begin with one
changed cell, clone up into a large mass, and remain localized.
The cells are very cohesive, so the tumor stays as a clump, yet at
some stage a cell slips out. Why? We don't know. Professor
Peter Alexander of the Chester Beatty Institute said simply, "It
is all jolly complicated." He is very intrigued by the possibility
that there is a relationship between the antigens on tumor cells
and their capacity to metastasize. A cell which has metastasized
carries the giveaway fingerprint on its surface and has done so
from the start. What Peter Alexander suspects is that a change
on even just the cell surface is potentially quite disastrous for
most malignant cells, for the immune system reacts to this
surface change. But *still* the cells find a way to evade the
immune system, and once they have done so, enhancing the
body's immune capacity may be no further use. For if the cell is
clever enough to do this, then it really doesn't make any

difference whether the patient's immune response is 50 or 100 percent efficient; the cell has already achieved its object.

One of the theories he and his colleagues at Chester Beatty are working on is that as the tumor's escape mechanism improves, so its metastatic capacity increases. A wart—a benign tumor—has a very poor "escape mechanism," but a widely disseminated tumor has a very good one. Some people believe, however, that it is an issue of sheer quantity, that immunological therapy is effective only when the cancer population is reduced to small amounts, like a few metastasizing cells. But spontaneous regression of tumors may kill this idea. For the fact remains that when spontaneous regressions occur they take care of large tumors as well as small ones, whether in animals or humans.

Peter Alexander has been looking into this question of tumor size experimentally, and has moved from mice to lambs. In a mouse the tumor is so large in relation to the animal that one can neither see nor analyze the biological processes. In sheep the relationship of tumor size to total animal mass is much more like that in man. But they have found some puzzling things. He and his colleagues have induced tumors in sheep by using a modified cat virus which causes leukaemia. When this is put into newborn lambs, the tumor appears about two weeks later, and is about one centimeter in size. The host reaction is very strong, yet the tumor grows and gets into a typical escape situation. Occasionally, though, and this happens with nearly half the experimental animals, when the tumor has grown for another two to three weeks and is nearly three times the original size, it suddenly disappears. They know this is due to an immunological reaction, but why doesn't the immune response, which certainly doesn't take more than a week or two to get under way, wipe out the tumor when it is small? Why the delay until it is that size? This is the kind of experimental evidence that may explode the myth of tumor size and immunological effectiveness. In all the years he has been working with cancer, Sir Alexander Haddow, one of the giants in cancer research, has never accepted this particular line. He has always said that if one could only find out why spontaneous regressions work, the mechanism would take care of large masses equally as well as small ones.

.   .   .

At the end of it all I pressed Avrion very hard, asking him to look on both sides of the immunological coin. "Be optimistic about cancer and cancer immunology," I invited him, "and then be thoroughly critical."

"There is not going to be any one scenario," he said. "There will be lots of alternatives. Immunotherapy is not a great white hope in itself. There will be many more immunotherapy trials in animals and man which will increase our understanding, possibly not so much in an empirical way, but in an inductive way. By using immunotherapy we will find out what makes immunotherapy work. Patients who by whatever means have been brought into some kind of remission will be plugged up with tumor antigens in the form of tumor cells, or other antigenic preparations, to prevent or delay the recurrence of the tumors.

"The other arm of the immunological approach to cancer, so far as it relates to the clinical side, is monitoring disease: finding the cancer area, being able to predict its course more accurately, monitoring the recurrences, monitoring the success of the immunotherapy programs themselves. All this will steam ahead. Many maneuvers which haven't yet been tried in man will be tried quite soon: taking out the lymphocytes, activating them and then putting them back; taking out the antigens and then adding bits and pieces on to the molecule; adding new determinants to them—perhaps viral determinants, created by mixing viruses and tumors. All this with the aim of encouraging the immunological response, making the lymphocyctes more aggressive and better at doing their job. So in ten years the situation will be *radically* changed for some cancers: probably for some of the leukaemias, radically changed for melanoma (a cancer of the skin which is a very nasty one indeed), and possibly for breast cancer too."

Then he reversed himself and showed me the other side of the coin. "Cancer immunology is a subject with which people have been 'messing around' for a long time. During the whole of this time, optimistic predictions have been made but have not been fulfilled, and at present, cancer immunology has very little to contribute. It contributes to monitoring in a very restricted way; this has nothing to do with cancer screening, but with predicting relapses and predicting metastases. As yet there is no cancer immunotherapy trial which has shown quite unequivocally that *any* success has been achieved by the immunological mechanism. The whole area needs a thorough going-over, not so much to establish the validity of any individual claim for a particular clinical success as to be critical about the *explanation* for that success. Where there has been a clinical success, however measured, following immunological therapy, the problem is to decide just how far the two are really related. One of the best trials was one in which Peter Alexander was involved, a trial on leukaemia at St. Bartholomew's Hospital. Patients with chronic myeloid leukaemia were first brought into remission by chemotherapy. If this was successful, the patients were then randomly assigned to either an immunotherapy program plus chemotherapy or a program for chemotherapy alone. The patients on chemotherapy alone always relapse, though they may take some time. The average time to relapse is on the order of half a year. The ones on the immunotherapy plus chemotherapy program are given drugs and the B.C.G. vaccine, plus some irradiated tumor cells. Now this is successful in that they *do* take longer before they relapse, doubling the time of remission. It is clear that the treatment is doing something. But what is not clear is whether the injection of the irradiated tumor cells with B.C.G. is operating in an immunological way. It might be doing something quite different. But this can be tested. It may well be, as Peter Alexander would argue, that the main effect of the immunotherapy is to reduce the level of blocking factors in the blood, and thus permit the normal response of the body via the T lymphocytes to take effect. This is an immunological explanation, of course, but what it may be telling us is that immunotherapy may work in a far more complicated way than we first thought."

It would be very surprising if it did not. Explanations in science may have to be simple, though the phenomena rarely are, and the precision we seek is nearer our grasp. Indeed, as this book is being written, an announcement has come from the Pasteur Institute of Paris that Fauve and Jacob have discovered a substance manufactured by both embryonic cells and cancer cells, which prevents lymphocytes from functioning. This is a remarkable and potentially very valuable discovery. The excitement and interest shown by the press and the public when this was announced was understandably great, so much so that the

Pasteur Institute issued another press release cautioning that this discovery does not mark the end of the problem of cancer. A lot more basic research needs to be done, but the future is promising. "When we look back," Bob Good had said to me, "at what we do to cancer today, chopping it out, burning it out, poisoning it out, it will all seem so crude." The phagocytes are being stimulated as strongly as Sir Ralph Bloomfield Bonington could possibly wish. So, too, are those of us watching from afar.

5

CANCER AND DRUGS:
I WANT THE PLATINUM BLUES!

Stimulate the phagocytes. Drugs are a delusion.

—Sir Ralph Bloomfield Bonington
(*The Doctor's Dilemma,*
George Bernard Shaw)

AS FAR AS DRUGS ARE CONCERNED, Sir Ralph's view has been widely shared. Oliver Wendell Holmes suggested that the whole of our *materia medica* should be sunk to the bottom of the sea, for though the fish might suffer, mankind would be infinitely better off. There is good reason for this view. If we consider the battery of material on the pharmacist's shelf, ranging from simple aspirin to the most potent stimulants and depressants, we see a range of compounds, many of which are useless or redundant, and some downright dangerous. Ours is a drug culture. We have been brainwashed into believing in the infallible chemical cure, instantly available and instantly effective. Once again this attitude reveals our ignorance, both about the nature of illness and about the role of drugs. Scepticism and caution are justified, and the old medical aphorism "Either the disease will kill you or you will kill the disease" contains elements of good common sense. As sailors and seamen now have a category of disaster labelled "Radar Assisted Collisions," so doctors, too, have their index of technological advance in a new category of illnesses called "Diseases of Medical Progress."

Once again, though, cancer makes its own rules, both in the nature of the disease and in the efficacy of our therapy. Granted that there are a few cases of natural and spontaneous remission, it is nevertheless the greatest folly to rely on the body's defenses alone. Immunotherapy is merely the latest missile on the therapeutic front where radiation, surgery and drugs have been weapons for some time.

One can look at the story of any specific anticancer drug, or at the history of the whole field of chemotherapy, and find mirrored there not only the paradoxes of cancer but those of drug therapy at large. The goal of all therapy is precision, and exquisite precision, and the magic bullet has been for doctors what the philosopher's stone was for the alchemists. Ideally, Huxley's doctor should metamorphose into the expert operator who with the skill of a sharpshooter delicately picks off cancer cells one by one. However, once again it is salutary to remember just where we are. Sometimes things work and we have no idea why, for we know very little about the basic process involved: acupuncture is one example, the polio vaccine is another. The history of chemotherapy in cancer is a history of many things that have been tried and don't work at all, a few things that work just a little, and fewer still that work well. So in tracing the history of just one drug out of many that have been tried, I found myself threading my way through a web of theory and experiment, or moving in a maze of personalities and politics, as individual scientists brought the force of their ideas to react both on a problem and on each other.

When I come to write about the platinum blues, I am frustrated by my incapacity to write several things simultaneously, for the story must be told at several levels: the levels of research and of personalities, of clinical trials and personal and scientific communication, of international politics and of scientific politics. I first encountered those levels in April 1973 at an international conference in Oxford, entitled "Second International Symposium of Platinum Coordination Compounds in Cancer Research." The brochure that was sent out with my invitation had clearly been put together by someone with a flair for alliteration and finesse. Colored platinum, as was only appropriate, this noble document reflected a rich approach to a complex problem and also the vast wealth of the industrial sponsors; Englehard Industries in America and England; the Rustenburg Platinum Mines Ltd. from South Africa; Abbot Laboratories; Matthey Bishop, Inc., from America; and Kyowa Hacko Kogyo Co. Ltd. of Japan. It promised a rich vein of intellectual ore, for the sessions had such titles as "The Chemistry of Coordination Complexes," "The Interactions with Biomacro-Molecules," "Bacterial and Viral Tissue-Culture Studies." It promised tough and stimulating discussion from brilliant participants: Sir Alexander Haddow, past director of the Chester Beatty Research Institute, London; Drs. Drobnik and Svec from the Slovac Academy of Sciences in Czechoslovakia; Dr. Krakoff of the Sloan-Kettering Cancer Institute of America. The whole glittering panoply, set against the glorious backdrop of Wadham College, Oxford, stemmed from a small discovery some years back. A group of people from a variety of disciplines and countries had shown that certain platinum compounds had marked antitumor effects. The conference would be the occasion when, with other colleagues and clinicians, they would review the past and future promise of the drug and refine and hone their accumulated knowledge on the stone of objection and counterobjection.

To trace the events that proceeded the conference, one must follow two threads. One thread can be found in England in the person of Bob Williams of Wadham College and his one-time pupil, Andy Thomson, now at the University of East Anglia. The other has to be followed in America with Barney Rosenberg, a professor in the Department of Biophysics, Michigan State University, where Bob sent Andy to study for a while. Bob and Andy are inorganic chemists whose prime interest has always been this. Their role in this story illustrates better than anything I know the ways in which the various branches of science complement and reinforce one another. Someone else's work from a totally unrelated field can bear most exactly on your problem. Andy's skill in spectroscopy and chemical synthesis was at Barney's disposal at a very critical time. Equally, someone else's discovery can open up a totally different field for you. So though working with Bob on platinum compounds started Andy on the road to his present acknowledged expertise in platinum coordination complexes, Barney was the one who led Andy into biological problems. As Barney remarked, "Andy was the first to synthesize the drug and confirm its structure in relation to its antitumor action. He is the true discoverer and is entitled to establish the name for the whole field."

When Andy Thomson came up to Wadham College, Oxford, to read chemistry, Bob Williams had been there for some years as chemistry tutor. I was to meet many of Bob's pupils. He is a remarkable man and clearly a much-loved one. Enormous intellectual authority is combined with sympathetic warmth, and these two traits alone would be enough to attract the admiration of undergraduates. Though an enthusiastic scientist, he keeps his science very much in check, with a balanced view of the enterprise in relation to other important aspects of society. Andy still speaks of his tutorials with Bob as "an experience of a lifetime." "You write an essay and hand it in, and next day you go for the tutorial. You think you have understood the subject. You have studied it for a week and think you are clued up, but the first question he asks you completely demolishes you. Instead of telling you the answer, he spends the next hour reassembling the bits. He will go back right to the beginning, saying, 'Okay, let's ask you something you do know.' And he will go through it with you stage by stage and will finally ask the question he asked at the beginning, and this time you will see the answer. He teaches you to think—to develop a subject logically."

Bob Williams himself went up to Oxford in 1940, and became a Fellow of Wadham College in 1955. At that time biochemistry was almost exclusively concerned with organic molecules, although this was not true in the early part of the century. About 1920 the first scientist purified and crystallized a biological molecule, a catalyst, and it was found to contain no metals at all. So inorganic chemistry was quietly dropped from the biochemical curriculum, and it remained in limbo for forty years. The general view was that there was no point in studying anything inorganic in biology, and where these substances appeared in biochemical preparations, they were considered impurities. The importance of the rare elements in organisms is a late discovery—Bob thinks it a puzzlingly late one.

Our theory of evolution presupposes that living materials have come from organic matter, which in its turn must have been derived from simpler inorganic compounds. Evolution is a drive toward complex structures and increased chemical efficiency. An organism will be able to capture from nature those substances which gives it biochemical advantage. Because of the close links between our environment and the forms of life on earth, those substances which an organism needs in the largest amounts are likely to be those which are present in the largest amounts. Substances like metals that are present only in small amounts will be utilized very selectively and with great sensitivity. Certain marine animals, the tunicates, accumulate vanadium; some nuts from Brazil contain barium; many rare metals such as chromium are found in the human body. These three metals are all absolutely essential in the particular organisms in which they occur, though we don't know their function. Bob Williams was looking for something to unify his work, so he thought he would study the functions of metals in biological systems. He went to see one of the giants in the biochemical field, to discuss the whole problem, but Bob's reasoning was dismissed with the comment that the metals were just impurities in his preparations. Bob wasn't convinced, however.

His contact with Barney Rosenberg came not through platinum molecules but through a shared interest in photosensitive molecules, molecules affected by energy from light. Bob had been looking at one of the most photosensitive of all, chlorophyll, a molecule which has an inorganic metal base, magnesium. As he was studying the photo-response of these molecules and that of various platinum compounds, Rosenberg was doing the same thing with the compounds that make up the pigments of the eye. They met first in Oxford, then again in California. Then Barney wrote and asked Bob to act as a scientific consultant for his platinum research, particularly with regard to cancer. Bob very happily agreed and made himself available from time to time to comment and advise on the work, when the whole group came together.

Meanwhile Andy Thomson was at Oxford doing his doctorate

with Bob. He started out on a straightforward problem in inorganic chemistry: trying to develop a piece of apparatus that would measure the energy of colored molecules. When you test an apparatus, you don't start with a most complicated problem or the most complicated molecule, but look around for some simple system, so Bob gave him some platinum compounds with rather unusual colors. They had a structural relationship to chlorophyll, and some of them responded to light, too. By the time the last year of work on his doctorate had arrived, he was both something of an expert in spectroscopy and, to use his own words, "pretty cheesed off with just measuring platinum things." From the distance of years he now admits what Bob Williams knew all along. It was time to move. Oxford had been rather inhibiting: it cosseted one too much. The problems had been too neat, were expected to be too neat. It was time, Andy recalls, to break out of a comfortable existence and learn just what the hard world was all about.

Bob knew that magnesium deficiency caused bacteria to elongate from a rod shape into a filamentous form. He also knew that Barney had observed that some reverse platinum complexes caused the same change. They differed sharply about the interpretation of this, but the observation was crucial for the story. At that time, Andy felt it to be one of the most exciting observations he had ever read about. He is still unable to analyze why, even though cell division is still a marvellous problem and platinum still a marvellous tool to study it. He already had a hankering to look at biological systems, partly because of Bob Williams' influence, so Barney's interest in both visual pigments and platinum directed him almost inevitably towards Michigan State University. There had been other offers—some very prestigious ones, from Yale, Harvard and the University of California—but it didn't weigh with him all that much, partly, he now suspects, because prestige was already so built into the system at Oxford that he both discounted it and was insulated from it. So Andy went to Michigan and Barney Rosenberg.

The contrasts between the two places and the two men could not have been greater. The one was initially a land-grant college; the other is one of the oldest universities in the world. I can think of only two characteristics common to East Lansing and

Oxford: The landscape is more or less flat and the sky tends to be gray. As if in compensation for Oxford's beautiful buildings, though, there is a spaciousness about Michigan which, when the sun shines, gives rise to most wonderful skyscapes, like those Eisenstein filmed in *Alexander Nevsky*. But if Oxford and East Lansing have two characteristics in common, Bob and Barney Rosenberg have only one—and that is science.

To meet Barney Rosenberg, to argue with him, is to meet and argue with an enthusiast. His ideas are presented rapidly, with an overwhelming authority and stunning force. A burst of eloquent fact precedes a battery of argument coming at you with such speed that the total effect is both overwhelming and dangerously convincing. One has to be very careful. I last saw him in his laboratory at M.S.U. during the coal miners' strike in England, but this was a problem which, one way or another, he was well on the way to solving. He has some bacteria which are blue and eat coal, and as they eat they produce a form of natural gas. So Barney, with characteristic breadth of vision—sweeping aside all difficulties, financial and engineering; ignoring all facts, economic and political—told me of his new, modern way to extract coal and even illustrated it with a most convincing diagram on his blackboard. In the future there will be no strikes, no horrible working conditions, no silicosis—all because of his blue bacteria. By the time he was finished, I was almost ready to invest in his scheme. His favorite aphorism, from Einstein, is "Nature is subtle, but not devious." This illustration encompasses the essence of the man. All science is really quite simple. In fact, as Barney speaks, *everything* seems simple.

The source of this simplicity is quite clear to Barney. Schrodinger's book *What is Life?* had the most marked influence on his scientific life, and he still speaks of it with shining admiration. Schrodinger admitted ignorance in biology, but used the theoretical arguments of physics to come to a most far-reaching and significant conclusion: the gene is a molecule, and therefore the only problem is to decide just what kind of molecule it is. This kind of logic was elementary and powerful, and logic of this form is a tool that Barney relies on a great deal. Many other people think, as I do, that simple logic can be totally misleading at times, but Barney is not convinced. For like many other physicists coming to biology he believes that the subject is not really that complex, and ultimately, in all its facets, it will yield to physics.

One feels that he chooses problems as exercises for his imagination, to give it scope and freedom. He is at the other end of the spectrum from those scientists who are happiest when following the smallest detail as it leads bit by bit through minute and exact ramifications into a total answer. Like Joyce Cary's character Gulley Jimson, he has to paint broad canvases, and like Gulley Jimson he pays a price for this in attitudes and achievements. Science demands wild heterodoxy and needs the men who walk alone as well as the more cautious experimenters but these men take gambles. In the end they are just as likely to be wrong as right; and until they are *proved* right, they risk not being taken seriously or even being isolated.

It is not just the force of simple logic which drives him, nor the usual desire among scientists to be first with ideas, but something else very personal and fundamental in his nature. He thrives on, insists on, a greater degree of freedom than the discipline and the community of science permits. "Freedom of speculation" is a favorite phrase of his, untrammelled by *anything*. He feels that scientifically this derives from his background in physics. He often speaks of speculations in physics which, so long as they are fruitful, are also allowed to be wrong. He doesn't even mind if he is wrong. It gets him into trouble, but he says, "I am willing to be led into trouble because I do not make my home in any one scientific dogma."

He has always been a scientific radical, both in the forms of his scientific theories and in his professional attitudes. He will not join any one scientific group. He steadfastly refuses to be a member of any scientific society because he feels that these associations tend to harden the arteries, to canalize the thought. If I want to provoke him, and I often do, with my talk about new social imperatives in science to which the profession must respond, I just insist that society should have a far greater say in the direction of science than it presently does. He always reacts instantly and strongly, for that way, he believes, lies scientific fascism. Any direction, any control, might fetter the imagination he prizes so strongly.

After getting his doctorate, Barney began to study visual pigments, looking at the efficiency of natural organic molecules as light conductors. This had been done before with photosynthetic pigments, but not with pigments in the eye. His first experiment was almost too successful, for he had no trouble in finding the effect he was looking for. If other people never accepted the "Rosenberg theory of electronic conductivity in visual receptors" that inevitably followed the easily acquired results, the empirical findings nevertheless were an important acquisition for his scientific store.

Short of having a scientific diary of the kind kept by Johann Kepler, one cannot know exactly what occurs and when in science. So it is difficult to locate the point at which cancer first came into Barney's mind and therefore into this story. He recalls looking at pictures that classical biologists draw of dividing cells. They looked not unlike dipole electric or magnetic fields, and he wondered whether there was anything electromagnetic about the process of cell division. There is absolutely no reason why there should be, and the answer is probably not, but it is the kind of jump in reasoning that he so often takes. A physicist—as Barney was then—looking at the visible pattern in cell division could say, "I'll pour some energy in. If I tickle the antennae of the dividing cell with energy at just the right frequency, it might pick up this energy and the division process would be altered. If different types of cells have different frequencies, then all I need to do is to find the right one and destroy the cell." In this way one could affect cell growth or cell division with an electric field. Such an idea might well never have occurred to a pure biologist.

In 1962, Loretta van Camp, with an extensive background in bacteriology and microbiology in the Michigan Public Health Service, came to work with Barney. She remembers that at her interview Barney discussed an experiment he wanted them to do. They would give short bursts of electrical current into a system of cultured bacteria to see if it affected the rate at which bacteria were produced. He mentioned cancer, too. Similar sorts of experiments had been done using that old bacteriological war-horse *E. coli*, but the only modification Barney proposed to make would be to use platinum electrodes. *E. coli* divides once every thirty minutes, so in twenty-four hours it goes through forty-eight divisions. The electricity would pulsate through, and if the electric current had any effect on bacterial divisions, that effect would be amplified as the whole system went through forty-eight generations of bacteria.

What happened then they both refer to as their "Eureka effect," for depending on the flip of a switch, there was an enormous difference. They turned on the current and the density of bacteria fell; they turned it off and the cell division increased again. Not only was cell division greatly modified, but enormous long filaments of bacteria were formed. From being short, tight little nuggets, they changed into a kind of bacterial vermicelli. Though cell division had ceased, growth was going on still, and the next problem was to find out why.

One can cover the whole of the next few months in a few sentences, though one inevitably diminishes the amount of work and the tightness of the proceedings. Obviously, it would have been sloppy to conclude from that experiment alone that electric currents cause bacterial growth to stop. So by switching a whole set of parameters—by trying electrodes of different metals—they were finally able to pinpoint the cause. Electricity had, in fact, very little to do with it. As one of Barney's colleagues, Tom Krigas, showed, there was contamination from the platinum electrodes, for as the current flowed, the metal reacted with the medium in which the bacteria were growing. They tried to reproduce the effect by putting standard platinum salts into the bacterial medium instead of passing an electric current through it, but nothing happened. So the platinum compounds in solution were just left on the shelf, but one day, testing them casually as she did from time to time, Loretta van Camp found that they now would cause filamenting. So by accident Barney realized that a photosensitive reaction was involved: light was altering the platinum compounds to an active form. In very low concentrations, about ten parts per million, the platinum formed a neutral compound with ammonia and chlorine, and this produced the filamentous effect. This was the compound that Andy Thomson was later to synthesize for Barney.

"Chance favors the prepared mind" is a well-known aphorism in science. This is one of the most important morals these experiments illustrate. For it was quite by chance that Barney was using platinum electrodes. Any other metal, and he would not have got the same effect. It was chance too that revealed a photosensitive reaction: the accident of leaving platinum solutions on the shelf in the light provided the clue as to what might be the active form. In fact, chance played such a large part in this story that Barney now says, somewhat wryly, that he would hate his scientific reputation to rest on his platinum work alone. Whenever the team came up against a "problem wall," a lucky accident or a chance finding helped them over it. On the other hand, he is being unduly modest about his own scientific strengths, for his mind was prepared for the unexpected finding—in this case, the filamentous growth of bacteria. Other people might have ignored the effect, but Barney Rosenberg did not. In addition, he had gathered about him some very astute colleagues from other disciplines: Gerry Drobnik, a microbiologist, who pointed out to Barney that the filamenting was of a most unusual form, and Scarlett Reslova, who worked out much of the biochemical detail. But the clear-cut logic and wide-ranging imagination made up Barney's particular strength and contribution.

Loretta van Camp recalls the day vividly. She is a dignified, almost subdued person, and yet the excitement still bubbles from her when she speaks. She remembers looking at the filamenting, turning to Barney and saying, "Isn't this what cancer's all about? Isn't this what we are after? For if you can stop a single bacterium from dividing, then why not a cell?" This unusual filamenting of bacteria finally pushed Barney Rosenberg in the direction of platinum as a possible anticancer drug. Apparently what had set him off was an article written in 1950 by Lwoff, an eminent French microbiologist, who pointed out that you could classify chemicals according to their effect on mammalian cells. Some are mutagenic—that is, they cause an irreversible change in the genetic make-up of the cell; some are carcinogenic, causing mammalian cells to become cancerous. Others produce a filamentous effect in bacteria, and still others cause the bacterial cell to lyse—that is, they disrupt the cell membranes so that the contents of the cell burst through. All these are the results of some kind of biochemical stress and strain. Now Bob Williams still feels that to draw a close parallel between these four phenomena was to push one's scientific luck much too far. He was adamant in telling Barney that a growth of this kind was really no clue to anything, certainly not a clue to cancer. But Barney proceeded on his own way. It is hard to know precisely what his logic was, but it probably went something like this: "I am interested in cell growth. Cancer is one form of cell growth and division. The question is, can I control it? I have by accident found a way to both control cell growth and stop cell division by using platinum compounds, so perhaps I can control growth of cancer cells in the same way as I can control it in bacteria. I will have a shot at it." He did and it worked. It is very likely that those who knew the cancer field well—Sir Alexander Haddow, for example—wouldn't have followed this path at all, indeed couldn't have followed this path, for they would know that *many* compounds cause filamenting (penicillin is one of them), but these substances have no effect on cancer cells at all. Trying platinum on cancer cells could possibly only have occurred to somebody who had growth at the center of his mind, not cancer. Perhaps it is not unfair to say that a somewhat naïve view of cancer led Barney Rosenberg to put the two things together. His gamble paid off, but some people thought him wildly optimistic, if not crazy.

To begin with, Andy Thomson was one of them, and now, in 1974, he is refreshingly honest about his first reactions both to the United States and to Barney Rosenberg. It is easy to visualize the tall, gangling figure, turning up at that vast university campus of forty thousand students, everything so totally different and unfamiliar to him. As so many of us did the first time in the States, Andy went, in his own words, "through an awful dip of 'It's the wrong decision.' " From England he had flown to the East Coast first and had stopped over to see a friend at Yale University. There was a party for the chemistry department that night, and the friend had invited him to come along. They were writing out name tags, and he asked, "What shall I write?" Immediately the answer came back: "Don't write M.S.U. Write Oxford: it's much better." It was unsettling. The harsh world was hitting out immediately as the bald facts of academic prestige, jealousy and prejudice surfaced.

His first encounter with Barney did nothing to restore his confidence. Andy remembers the experience vividly. He was picked up at Lansing Airport and taken straight to the lab. It was Saturday afternoon, and no one else was there. Theirs is not a luxurious lab—few of the scientists' laboratories that I visited are—but they walked around it and Barney was enthusing all the time about his ideas and his problems. Andy's spirits slowly began to sink as he reacted to these crazy problems, which were not being tackled in the way he would have tackled them. Filamentous growth and cancer, an unlikely theory of vision and photoconductivity—it all seemed so speculative. The enthusiasm and ideas must have poured over him like a waterfall, leaving him drenched and without secure footing. He got to his hotel and sat in his room, struggling with himself, for his Yale friend had offered him a job, with a nice, neat, solid little problem to be solved on platinum. It was the first time he had ever left Europe, and that night a neat scientific problem represented security. He almost picked up the phone and said, "I'll come."

But he stayed and things changed and Andy changed, though it took a long time. In many ways he feels he didn't find himself until two years later, when he finally had his own lab at the University of East Anglia in England and began doing things his own way. He came to admire so many things about Barney—the way in which he would analyze problems, for one. He was provoked and stimulated, for an extreme enthusiast becomes an extreme irritant, if only because one has to prove him wrong. So he spent hours in the library digging out facts and reading widely in an effort to show Barney the holes in his rarefied logic. Andy says he has never read so much as he did in those two years. Bob Williams, his teacher, was also capable of launching off on a novel tack, but he would read carefully and take off from what was known. Barney would take up from a hunch.

Another thing Andy came to admire was Barney's capacity to do different things. So many people in science do one kind of experiment for their doctoral dissertation and then go on doing the same sort of experiment for the next fifty years. Scientists even admit this about themselves. They take the next obvious compound off the shelf and do to that new compound whatever measurement their expertise dictates. But not Barney. He will say, "I'm going to attack the vision problem," or, "I'm going to attack the cancer problem," or "I'm going to attack the aging problem." He insists on choosing a complex problem to be solved, and though the odds are that he may not solve it at all, he refuses to be constricted in any way, most of all by himself. Andy Thomson admired that greatly.

Besides the contrast between the two towns and the two men, there was the contrast, equally great, between the ambience of the two universities. Oxford can be very overpowering for a young man. People are very bright, and competition is stiff. A student may not only fail to thrive, but at the end of his time may come to have a completely false idea of his own capacities, even underestimating them. This happened to Andy. He needed to go to M.S.U. to find himself and gain confidence, and Barney provoked him into the best work he could. The two years had "one hell of an impact"!

Andy worked on two problems at Michigan: the visual pigments and the platinum problem. With the platinum problem, he was trying to find out exactly what was in the soup that the bacteria were growing in. Was there one platinum compound or were there many? The soup had to be taken apart chemically, so he separated it and found there was a neutral complex of some rather special platinum compounds. He and Barney submitted for publication the paper announcing their results, and the referees commented that it was fine, but it would be even better if they inverted the experiment in order to confirm the point doubly. What they had to do was synthesize suspected critical compounds, feed them to the bacteria, and see if these compounds also induced the filamentous growth. There were two active compounds of platinum that were likely candidates: cis compounds and trans compounds, which differ only in the position of the chlorines. There was no way to tell which of the two present in the soup was the active complex, so Andy Thomson made them both and they were both tested. The cis forms, with two chlorine atoms next to each other on the molecule instead of opposite each other, were the important ones for inducing the filamentous effect.

At this point Andy remembers hearing the first suggestion about cancer. During the time he had been there, little had been said about it, but he was told that Barney was going to get hold of some white mice with tumors and inject platinum solutions into them. The laboratory personnel were apparently somewhat less than enthusiastic. It seemed ridiculous, though not necessarily for scientific reasons. No logic led one to suppose that it *would* work or that it wouldn't. There was no theory, or precious little theory, on which to base the experiment. It seemed a typically extravagant American idea, injecting many dollars' worth of platinum into white mice, and jokes about platinum mice were tossed around about as freely as Barney's ideas. There was also lots of red tape, not to mention the technological difficulties of keeping animals in a laboratory where no animals had ever been used before. They all tried to dissuade Barney, but of course they couldn't. In September 1967, the point at which Andy was returning to England, the first cages of white mice arrived.

He heard nothing from Barney for a whole year, and everything seemed to have died down. Then one day the mail brought him a manuscript; the paper on the work which was to be published in *Nature*. Written on the corner of this manuscript were a few simple words: "Hold onto your hat, Andy, these may be the best anticancer drugs yet. Barney."

They aren't yet, for the results are still inconclusive, but in the intervening year Barney had done just what he said he was going to do. From Professor Beneke, who had been working with a mushroom extract which had some antitumor activity, Barney had obtained a group of mice that had solid tumors, and used them to test some of the platinum complexes. Loretta went over to Professor Beneke's lab to learn the drug techniques and find a dosage level of platinum solution that the animals would tolerate. She then went through the standard procedure, the protocol of the National Cancer Institute that gives the routines necessary for testing a new drug by injection in animals. Eight to ten days after the injections, the tumors were regressing. She says, "I just went off the floor with excitement." They repeated the procedure three times in some twelve to twenty animals, and by using the synthesized material which Andy had made up for them just before he left, got 100 percent positive inhibition of the tumor every time.

This was in June 1968. When Barney felt really secure with his discovery—a novel, inorganic complex that exhibited antitumor activity against a tumor which was notoriously drug-resistant—he contacted the National Cancer Institute and spoke to Dr. Gordon Zubrod, in charge of chemotherapy testing. He was invited to go down and give a talk, so he went to Washington with four different samples of the platinum chemical and talked about the research to a small group of people. These were mostly directors of the research section, and the first response was, he remembers, one of total disbelief. Their attitude wasn't the result of sheer obscurantism, for not only were his findings totally unexpected, but there were also some rather strong theoretical reasons why heavy metals were considered to be most unsuitable candidates for an anticancer drug. However, by law the institute is required to test any drug or chemical that any reasonable scientist sends in to them, so even if they didn't like the idea they still had to test the sample. Sensing their lack of enthusiasm, Barney left the material behind and returned to East Lansing. Two months later and well into the fall, he telephoned and asked if they had had any results. They finally called back with the news they had had quite positive results on a leukaemic tumor, L1210, their standard screening tumor. As a consequence, the M.S.U. Department of Biophysics finally got a cancer grant to develop the research into the drug.

The paper was published in *Nature*. The National Cancer Institute did their tests and everything could have simmered along quietly. Platinum might have turned out to be—as it may well still turn out to be—just one of a number of drugs which are being tried. Admittedly, it was more striking than most: in mice it was clearly active against a very resistant tumor, and also effective against a broad range of tumors. In rats the drug's effect was so potent that the animal could survive to the day before expected death, and after injection, the tumor would regress so completely that the animal would survive. These effects were not totally unusual, however. What was unusual was that this occurred with a heavy metal.

Scientific results not picked up by scientists, to be repeated and extended, are lost forever. They never even get into the mainstream of scientific life. But it makes a great deal of difference just who picks them up and repeats and extends them. Barney Rosenberg is the first to admit that he was extremely lucky. No wild enthusiasm was generated in his own country, but from England came the kind of response he wanted. A few months after the article had appeared in *Nature*, he received a letter from Sir Alexander Haddow, then director of the Chester Beatty Institute for Cancer Research, the most prestigious of the English cancer institutes. Alexander Haddow wrote that he had read the paper with the greatest interest, since he had always felt that platinum in some compound or other should show antitumor activity.

It is interesting to ask why. Rosenberg had no previous experience and very little theory to go on when he made the decision to try this drug against tumors, but Alexander Haddow could be expected to have solid reasons. In this case, it was just one more of his aphorisms: "That which causes cancer can also cure it."

If cancer is a defect in molecular machinery that causes one cell to behave aberrantly, then we must find a drug to either kill the cell or divert it. We are looking for molecular wrenches to throw in the works, substances which can mess up the molecular mechanism. Certain metals are known to be carcinogens, since by interfering with the basic processes, they cause cancer; therefore, by theoretical inversion, the injection of metals into the organism should also interfere with a cell's molecular mechanism and so help cure cancer. This is crude and imprecise, but so is the general rationale behind cancer drug action.

Many years ago, the International Nickel Company sent Sir Alexander Haddow a series of platinum compounds, but he got no positive results from testing them. After reading the Rosenberg paper in *Nature*, however, he immediately had the company synthesize the same compounds that Rosenberg had been using. He tried them out in a series of experiments, confirmed the work, and then wrote to Rosenberg. Barney came to London and gave a seminar where a number of people from the Chester Beatty, including Dr. Tom Connors, were present; Haddow in his turn visited the laboratory at M.S.U., and in this way the expansion of the work was sparked, both with regard to research and clinical trials. Barney says now, "I suspect that Haddow's interest was the greatest contribution to the development of the field. It would have grown without it, but at a much slower pace. His interest sparked the interest of a large number of others, and his reputation carried it along to a degree that no one else could have achieved. Obviously, in the field of cancer research I am a nonentity, and certainly on the basis of my work alone, and on the basis of the fact that it was such a novel thing, it could have sunk among the empirical data of all the other anticancer drugs."

The National Cancer Institute of America finally took an interest, not only because they had found anticancer activity in the drugs, but also for a reason which they were only later to admit to Barney. They were tired of having the same old chemicals, with minor modifications, come back to them time after time. They and their counterparts at Chester Beatty are always looking for new classes of compounds which will show antitumor activity in the hope that a major breakthrough will occur. Certainly, these platinum compounds had the merit of novelty, opening up a whole new area of chemistry for chemotherapists, and also, incidentally, for chemists themselves. Thus under the effective catalytic action of Haddow's interest, this rather unusual compound went into clinical trials both in America and in England.

I discussed the first results from England with Dr. Tom Connors of the Chester Beatty Institute, and Dr. Eve Wiltshaw, a clinical oncologist at the Royal Marsden Hospital, London. These are two of the people who would now take the antitumor drug to the next stage, from the laboratory to the patient. Tom is a big, burly man with auburn hair. He occupies a very small room in the Chester Beatty Institute, in the Fulham Road, where he works against the counterpoint of traffic noise. The whole atmosphere in his laboratory is one of relaxed but hard effort, in a situation where there is neither time nor money for glamour. The scientific bandwagon never picked up his generation—as of course it passed by many English scientists—for the show really only got on the road as "big time" in the United States in the 1950's and 1960's. His room is small, but there is a second desk in it anyway, which is occupied by Peter, his technician. The laboratory is off this office, and there is much activity and movement between the two all the time. Just as the Sloan-Kettering Institute has a close attachment to Memorial Hospital, so the Chester Beatty Institute is closely attached to the Royal Marsden next door, and the scientists have an equally good working relationship with the clinicians there. It doesn't take more than three minutes to know that Tom is a man who knows what he's talking about, who has seen all these things before but knows that genuine progress is being made.

One of the things he likes about the platinum story is how well it illustrates many of the principles of scientific discovery—for instance, the recognition of the chance findings. As Tom said, "It is no good making an observation unless you are clever enough to realize what you've done." The platinum story also illustrates for him other important morals that relate particularly to the problem of anticancer drugs. First, one never knows what may happen. He told me what I hadn't known, that the platinum compound in question had been in chemistry textbooks since the 1870's. It was known as Peyrone's chloride, but nobody had suggested that it should be tested as an antitumor agent because there was no reason to believe that it would be effective. Once the compound had been tested, however, there was immediate interest all over the world, and at Chester Beatty, they were encouraged, even pressured, into trying it. Dr. Wiltshaw admitted that Alexander Haddow really pushed them. Their own reluctance came from an a priori conviction that it would turn out to be just like all other cytotoxic agents.

Once they tested it, the second moral surfaced, which is that a whole battery of problems will always arise, and there is no way of avoiding them. Sulphonamide drugs, for instance, are very selective against certain bacteria. Even a very low dose will destroy the infecting organisms, while a high dose will not kill the patient; with the so-called cancer therapeutic agents, however, the dose which destroys a tumor cell is very close to the dose that kills a patient. Therefore, there will always be serious side effects of one sort or another.

All people in all clinics who use anticancer agents are in effect using poisons, and the reason they use them is that the tumor is more dangerous to the patient than the poison. Used under the right conditions, you get some benefits, though it may be very difficult to get the right conditions. But at the same time the drugs have all sorts of toxicity, for since all cancer drugs interfere with DNA, they affect *every* dividing cell in the body. For a start, they will affect the blood cells, and the patient may well get anaemia.

The pattern is always the same. A new drug is discovered and everyone gets excited. The drug goes for clinical trial, and then everyone gets upset, because it is toxic in one way or another. In the case of the platinum compound, it was kidney toxicity. Suddenly, all the excitement which has been developed damps down because of the severe side effects. The work goes in cycles. Scientists discover a compound; industrialists develop it; doctors place it into clinical trials; problems arise. The drug becomes less interesting and everybody becomes gloomy. Then a new compound comes by and they all get excited again.

Consequently it is very important, Tom emphasized, to keep very level-headed about these drugs. Our models are not very predictable and while we may have the most magnificent antitumor agents in animals, with one type of agent specifically inhibiting one type of tumor, nobody in chemotherapeutic research ever believes he or she will discover the one universal anticancer agent. The reason is simple: we don't even know the differences between cancer cells and normal cells yet. Researchers do know that given the right conditions—and in that phrase a multitude of problems and assumptions is hidden—and given even just one difference between a tumor cell and a normal cell, we can exploit that difference and get regression of the tumor. Selectivity is possible, but only for one class of tumor at a time. But in cancer we have many hundreds of types of malignant cells, all with different biochemical characteristics. An agent which can cure one type of malignant cell will not necessarily have any effect whatsoever on another type.

Tom also insisted that while we must be realistic we needn't be pessimistic. He was merely emphasizing how little we really know about cells. There are undoubtedly differences between the normal and malignant cells, and eventually we will find out what these are; in some cases we have already done so. When we have that knowledge, then we can exploit it in our therapy.

Another problem with cancer drugs is the constant fact that no animal tumor prescribes for a human tumor. If we knew, for example, that carcinoma of the large intestine in the mouse told us something really genuine about carcinoma of the large intestine in man, then scientists would have a field day. They could spend five million dollars screening all the compounds in the world against that particular carcinoma in mice, and if they found a good compound, they could go straight into man. As it is, if they pick up one that works in animals, then they know this is just the start of their efforts. This is depressing, but it is part of the research to get new and effective compounds. These almost always come as a result of a chance discovery or a screening program. They are not found by search based on a purely scientific rationale because the fundamental knowledge is not yet there.

With chemotherapy, we are working not so much at the frontiers of knowledge as at the frontiers of ignorance. We know so little about what is going on, and we are debarred by the very nature of the disease from doing a proper scientific experiment which would help our understanding. When new classes of compounds with antitumor effects are discovered, we cannot know how they work unless they are put into patients. In effect, we are putting them into patients *before* we know how they work. We must do this partly because they *might* be wonder-drugs and partly because we are left in a totally static situation if new agents are not tried. At the beginning, however, for the sake of the patient, new, untried drugs cannot be used in preference to those whose effects are known. Therefore, they are given only to patients in critical situations.

This presents another problem, for leaving aside the human aspect for the moment, even if the patient does live as a result of the treatment, it is almost impossible to make any theoretical deduction from the situation. In a situation involving a large tumor, a critically ill patient, and a new drug, the dice are really loaded against a genuine inference. A paradox has arisen; as Dr. Wiltshaw pointed out to me, the more drug therapy progresses, the more complicated its analysis becomes. In the days when there was practically no drug therapy at all, the tendency was not to treat those patients in whom the cancer started to spread. But if a patient did come to the cancer wards of a hospital like Marsden, instead of being sent home to die, then one had an untouched patient so far as drugs were concerned. Thus whatever effect the treatment produced, one could deduce that the drug had something to do with it. Now, however, patients with cancer go through a series of drugs, and it is difficult to say with any conviction that what has occurred is really the results of the last drug given. Thus a doctor must be governed by the fact that the drug he is now going to try does present some potential over and above the ones they are already offering, but to test this potential he can only plan fairly small changes in drug dosage, watch for the effects and try to build up some picture of drug action. It is all rather unsatisfactory, but until we know more, we have no alternative.

In almost every one of these respects, the story of the platinum compounds so far has recapitulated the story of almost every other effective known anticancer agent. There are only about thirty of these agents from the thousands of compounds which have been screened. In mice, the platinum compounds were wonderful. They were broad-spectrum agents—that is, active against almost every type of tumor. In man, they are effective only against one or two tumors. In mice, there were no side effects. In man, high doses of the platinum compounds have raised severe problems of kidney poisoning, and this will be their limiting factor. Kidney toxicity is rare, and under these circumstances doctors are very careful. If the platinum drug had turned out to be the wonder drug, people would have been delighted but they would have also been astonished. As it is, the future of the first drug is in a critical phase. It is too good to abandon, but not good enough to extend. The fact that the very first drug was not as effective in patients as in mice was disappointing but understandable and inevitably diminished the enthusiasm of the clinicians, for the most important factor in the acceptance of a drug is enthusiasm for it from the people who have to administer it. The scientists are now at work on several new aspects of the platinum compounds. There is not just one drug now, for Barney's group has developed a whole new class of interesting drugs—the blues. Whereas the first ones were lemon-yellow, the second group showed a whole spectrum of color from light-blue to deep cobalt. Barney is hopeful that the results from these will exceed the very best trial of the first compounds, in which seven of fifteen American terminal patients with testicular tumors have had complete remissions. In England, there were four complete remissions of the thirty-five terminal cancer patients with ovarian cancers that had been totally unresponsive to other cancer drugs. These are small figures, but the nature of the problem is such that we have no right to expect miracles.

The difference between the first and second generation of the platinum compounds lies not only in their changed color and in their chemical structure, but in their effects on animals. So far in animals the blues do not produce the same degree of kidney poisoning, and this means that higher dosages can be given. Barney Rosenberg is now extremely cautious in extrapolating from the animal situation to the human situation, however, especially as the Chester Beatty people have not yet duplicated his results. He is rightly cautious, since his own direction of work may well be changed by this situation. If the platinum blues show the same kinds of limiting toxicity that was present in the first generation of drugs, then the enthusiasm for platinum may diminish to the vanishing point and he might as well drop the subject. But if the drugs do not produce kidney poisoning in humans, then he will have a remarkable success on his hands. The most pessimistic view, the thing that he constantly worries about, is that the drug will continue to do beautifully in animals, but, to use Barney's own words, "won't do a damn thing in humans whatsoever. And in that case there is nothing to it and we might as well forget the whole story. This is something we learn to live with, though it is a fear at the back of our minds all the time."

This would be a scientific sentence of death, but anyone who chooses to work with anticancer drugs learns to live with this sword of Damocles. These are the two extremes, though, and the drug will probably behave in a manner somewhere between them both.

Each of the people concerned in this story is developing the scientific ramifications in some direction or other. In Barney's lab they are now trying to synthesize and analyze the action of as many new variants of the drug as they possibly can, in an attempt to understand the relationship between the structures of these molecules and their biological activity. Therapeutically, they believe there could be many other applications of these chemicals for medical purposes, possibly as agents against viruses and bacteria. It looks as if they may also be useful in the treatment of arthritis, but all these applications have to be developed. Their research is now being financed by both the National Cancer Institute and the industrial platinum companies.

Tom Connors is, amongst other things, working on a drug

synthesized by Martin Tobes of University College, London. It is a platinum 11 complex, where the therapeutic index is something on the order of 500. The therapeutic index is defined as the dose which kills 50 percent of the animals divided by the dose that cures 90 percent of them. If the result of this division is 500, this means that you need a very large dose to kill, but only a small one to cure. The drug is so fantastically active against a tumor and does so little biochemical damage to an animal that—Tom quips—"you can almost let the animal smell the drug and it will be cured." This is a truly remarkable result. Something very precise is happening; the molecular wrench is being gently eased into the works rather than being thrown into the system. The drug has not yet been tried clinically, however, because it won't dissolve. You can put it into laboratory animals by mixing it with peanut oil so that it forms an opaque mess, but you can't put an opaque mess into human beings. The human protocols say that a new drug which is to be injected intravenously must have a particle size smaller than the smallest capillaries, so Tom Connors is trying to reduce the particles of this drug to a size of less than one micron.

Andy Thomson is pushing hard on the structure of platinum compounds in order to try to understand the exact mechanisms of their action. The difference between the two forms of platinum, the trans and the cis, lies—as I mentioned earlier—in the position of the two chlorine ions in the molecule. It is a mild difference, but a critical one. Apparently the two chlorine ions will float away if the compound is put in water. They are called the "leaving groups"; in the new platinum compounds, the leaving groups are different. In a paper written jointly with Bob Williams and Scarlett Reslova, who has now returned to the University of Prague, Andy speculated that the action of the platinum drug consists in picking up two or more groups from the DNA of the cancer cell. The distance between the bases in the DNA sequence is approximately the same as the distances between the two chlorine ions on the platinum molecule. Thus if the chlorine ions have floated away, the whole platinum molecule fits neatly into the DNA sequence, bridging the rungs of the ladder. When the DNA starts to unzip, separating in order to divide and replicate, the platinum molecule is in the way and the process is stopped.

But Barney Rosenberg isn't at all certain that this is the mechanism. He knows that the platinum does cause lesions in the DNA, though not lethal ones. But by making the tumor virus express itself and so form new proteins, it also increases the antigenicity of the cell, and he feels this is the critical effect. Once the antigenicity becomes increased, the body begins to recognize the tumor as foreign, and the immune system of the host finally kills it. It is not the drug then which kills the tumor cell, he argues, but the body itself. He believes that he now has fresh evidence for this. Using a new batch of platinum coordination compounds with a whole range of colors from blue to green, he has induced the formation of DNA particles on the cell surfaces of eighteen types of tumor. The presence of DNA in this position may well enhance the antigenicity of these cells.

When Tom Connors was talking to me about the pattern common to all drug discoveries, he turned to Peter, his technician, and said frivolously, "How many brilliant discoveries did *we* make last week?" Peter didn't hesitate for a moment: "Oh, about three, I should think." "But they don't last, do they?" "No, only for a day or so," Peter replied. Chemotherapy is a complex and difficult area. Most people in cancer chemotherapy are now trying theoretical models with animals and concentrating their efforts there. They transplant tumors and try all the elements that are at present available for the treatment of the cancer to see how effective these are. Genuine anticancer agents have been found only by people using animal models in this way; by now, of the thirty such compounds, five or six have come from the Chester Beatty Institute. Though the rate of discovery is certainly not three a week, it is nevertheless quite high, about three or four a year, but depressingly, as Tom pointed out, they tend to be the same. They are all cytotoxic; they all cause bone-marrow damage and other poisoning.

So, all over the field, scientists are moving into a new stage of research, on the basis of the knowledge that has so far been built up. More complex compounds are being tested in more complex models. If to the outsider the progress seems slow, it is because like all good scientists, they are walking before they run. With our present knowledge certain patients are being kept alive, and that is halfway to curing them. The right drugs, in the right location, in the right sequence, at the right dose level, at the right time, now have a 50 percent chance of producing a complete remission; ten years ago, the situation was very different. I once asked Barney Rosenberg an unfair question: if he or someone in his family had cancer, would he use his own drug? "Absolutely," he said, "with certain qualifications. Firstly, I would want to be given something which would stimulate the immune system of my body generally; then I would want the platinum blues, but the dose would have to be administered in one single day, spread out over twenty-four hours." Since the efficiency of a drug is affected by the time and manner of the administration, this would be for maximum impact. You can't say fairer than that.

As I walked through the quadrangle at Wadham on the last evening of the conference, I thought about doctors' dilemmas. Shaw was funny, but even in Sir Ralph's terms the germ of modern ideas emerges. "The phagocytes won't eat the microbes unless the microbes are nicely buttered for them," says Ridgeon, the central figure. But drugs cannot be total delusions, then, for how, I wondered, do you butter microbes or tumors except with a drug. Barney believes that his drug, too, works partly by "stimulating the phagocytes." He may be right: anyway, here we all were, because of his drug. A few years of solid work had brought eighty people together to Oxford for three days, and a few patients into remission in America and England, a pattern that is repeated whenever cancer drugs and chemotherapy are concerned. The rest of the story has yet to come.

6

CANCER AND POLITICS:
THE DEMANDING ART OF PATRONAGE

Is not a Patron, my Lord, one who looks with unconcern on a man struggling for life in the water, and when he has reached the ground, encumbers him with help?

—Samuel Johnson (Letter to Lord Chesterfield, 1754)

I WAS ENCUMBERED one morning with books and a tape recorder, so instead of walking up to the laboratories, I took a cab. Rye taxi drivers are generally subdued, but my driver must have strayed from his home territory, for he was the original Brooklyn cabby, delivering a rapid discharge of observations on the State of the Union, the World, the White House and God. As we waited at the lights to turn into the drive, he said, "Is it true that this here's a cancer place?" "Yes," I replied. "Are they working real hard?" he inquired. "Yes," I replied again, "it strikes me that they are working very hard." "But," he insisted, "are they making any discoveries?" "Yes," I said, "I'm sure they are." "Well, they'd better," he declared flatly. We drove through the gates and down to the front entrance in silence. I leaned through the window and settled up. "Why had they better?" I inquired. "Well, it's my money, isn't it?" he said, and drove away.

I was very thoughtful as I went into the hall, for it *is* his money—at least a great deal of it is—and he is supporting cancer research in many other countries besides America. The level of nurture has risen so fast that along with the advancing tide of discovery come such impish dicta as "More people are now living off cancer than ever died of it," and the one I was moved to coin, "If you haven't got cancer, then you're working on it." The statistics supplied by the National Cancer Institute, from the program for Annual Planning Project Requirements, are formidable. By July 1, 1975, it is estimated that 670,000 people in the United States will be working on cancer; 27.4 percent of them scientists; 14.1 percent research assistants; 14.9 percent technicians and 10.5 percent clerical staff. The clinicians *et al.* make up the rest. The budget for 1973, given to me by the financial management branch of the National Cancer Institute, indicates that in that year some 800 million dollars was spent on cancer research; 57.4 percent of this came from the National Cancer Institute, the remainder from private or other sources. Over the years the American Cancer Society, which began funding cancer research as far back as 1946, has also raised its commitment proportionately. For example, in its fiscal year 1973–74, it awarded 498 research grants to 127 major institutions and scientists, both American and foreign, at the cost of twenty-six and a half million dollars.

The commitment of the United States to this "biological moonshot" has brought other things besides money along in its wake: success and envy, achievement and frustration, an opportunity for good scientists but also one for entrepreneurs. The story behind the National Cancer Institute illuminates the whole question of the relation between the patronage of science and the pace, the content, indeed, the guarantees, of scientific discovery. Since the sums and the numbers of people in cancer research are now so vast, both the professionals and the society which supports them are being forced for the first time in their history into an examination of the nature of the social contract between them. The situation has reached its apogee in the United States, where King Midas has real gold in his coffers; but who shall have the gold and what the gold can guarantee are other questions.

A commitment to cancer in the United States was neither a

new idea nor a new undertaking when during 1970 momentum built up to culminate in the National Cancer Act of 1971. The origins of this activity can be traced back not to the aspirations of scientists, but to a highly charged appeal made to the Senate on May 18, 1928, by Matthew Neely, the senior Senator from West Virginia.

> I propose to speak of a monster that is more insatiable than the guillotine; more destructive . . . than the World War, more irresistible than the mightiest army . . . more terrifying than any other scourge . . . The monster . . . has infested and still infests every inhabited country; it has preyed and still preys upon every nation; it has fed and feasted and fattened . . . on the flesh and blood and brains and bones of men, women and children in every land. The sighs and sobs and shrieks it has exhorted from perishing humanity would, if they were tangible things, make a mountain. The tears it has wrung from weeping women's eyes would make an ocean. The blood that it has shed would redden every wave that rolls on every sea. The name of this loathsome, deadly and insatiate monster is, "cancer."

Reading this in our present, less emotional, climate, I have to confess that my immediate reaction was an irreverent "Sock it to 'em, Matthew!" for I have found it consistently difficult to adjust to such hyperbolic language. At the same time I was rather ashamed of this reaction. I have only to relive my hours with Rachel and Jan to appreciate the intensity of Matthew Neely's appeal. The successful outcome of such emotional appeals depends on the culture, and the reason why they are consistently present in the American scene, whether in Congress, the courts, or on Madison Avenue, is a good pragmatic one—they work. Indeed, Dr. George Mathé, one of France's most outstanding immunologists, has ruefully remarked that compared to his English and American colleagues, he has much more difficulty raising funds for cancer research in France. He believes this is due to the matter-of-fact manner in which the French treat cancer as just one disease among others, being as little or as much moved by appeals for financial support as they would be by appeals for new bridges across the Seine.

Matthew Neely's initiative culminated in the Neely Bill in the Senate, but his bill failed to pass in the House, and in a curious foreshadowing of what would happen in a similar situation forty years later, Neely lost his seat in the fall elections. But between the Cancer Act of 1928 and the National Cancer Act of 1971, many actions and thoughts were repeated—not just scenes of personal and political conflict, but struggles for power between scientists and politicians and between the executive and legislative branches. One basic question was: who was going to control scientific and medical research? By the early seventies it was at least clear who was *not* going to—namely, the political administration. From small beginnings in the thirties to the enormous expansion during the fifties and onwards, the policies and direction of National Institutes of Health were in the hands of scientist-administrators. In splendid isolation, the institute was internally operated, free of political influences, and to an extent insulated from gross political issues. To the scientists, this seemed not only terribly logical, but somehow fitting. In any case, during the postwar era the political issues were in good hands with such superb supporters and advocates in the Congress as Senator Lister Hill. There seemed no reason to modify policy. This state of affairs had gone on for so long that when congressional influence waned in the seventies and political battles moved closer and closer, the members of NIH were totally unprepared, let alone well versed. It is against this historical background that we must view the traumas that followed the passing of the National Cancer Act.

Many people were catalysts in galvanizing support and action during the three years' frenetic activity that preceded the passing of the present act. In varying degrees, and in a variety of ways, four were unusually significant; in this day and age it is highly appropriate that they were all women: Mary Lasker, Mathilde Krim, Anna Rosenberg Hoffman, and Ann Landers.

Mary Lasker has been involved in this story for a long time; indeed, she is a crucial character in the history of support for medical research in the United States. She is a woman of great compassion and of great energy, a "doer." The Albert D. Lasker Foundation for Medical Research, established by her and her husband, focuses its attention and income on basic science as the essential support underneath medical work and medical practice. She would have applauded T. H. Huxley's attitudes; she might even have given him a grant. I would characterize her as a "gutsy pragmatist"—combining compassionate emotional commitment with tough, practical realism and a sense of political clout. In the years between 1930 and 1969, she built herself a veritable fortress of experience, from which she sallied forth on various campaigns, with aides ranging from senators to lobbyists, from scientists to newspapermen. Her method of operation is very open, and she mobilizes powerful social and political forces with pinpoint accuracy, applying pressure to those few pivotal points which are likely to be vital to her concern. She uses her money and influence to further all those causes covered by the umbrella term "medical philanthropy," a field in which she is now a unique and remarkable figure. It is clear that having decided to focus one of her efforts on cancer, she would have a Plan—with a capital P—all ready from the beginning, with a list of people to approach figured out and the tactical moves decided.

One day in the spring of 1970, she telephoned a friend of hers, Dr. Mathilde Krim, a research biologist at Sloan-Kettering. Dr. Krim's husband, Arthur Krim, had been very active in various Democratic party and presidential campaigns, was a personal friend of Lyndon Johnson and had also been his special advisor at the White House on general affairs. Mary Lasker suggested to Dr. Krim that they go down to Washington to see Ralph Yarborough. The liberal Senator from Texas was running for reelection in the fall of 1970, and was facing severe political and financial problems in his campaign, for he had been amongst the earliest supporters for the rights of the Chicanos, and was meeting the predictable reactionary backlash from the conservatives in the state. The purpose of their visit was to persuade Yarborough to initiate support for cancer on a massive scale in Congress, for as Mary Lasker said, the existing level verged on the ridiculous. It was a deliberate choice. Ralph Yarborough was chairman of the Subcommittee on Health, and they hoped that if the bill became available, he would sponsor it in the Senate. He had been intrigued for some time by the promise of a marriage between cash and cancer research, after having heard the testimony of Dr. Lee Clark of Houston several years before, back in the golden days of money, science and politics. Dr. Clark's testimony took the form of an outright prophecy that ten years and ten billion dollars would "lick cancer."

Yet even before this, the American Cancer Society had realized the need for effort and had been an active agent for mobilizing congressional and public support. Since the early 1950's, in fact, they had been pounding away at Congress, partly through the person of Colonel Luke Quinn, a full-time lobbyist who acted as liaison officer between the society and the legislature.

Quinn understood the legislative process superbly, and it was Quinn who was now able to pull the required activity together, and who recognized that a panel of consultants would be necessary. Senator Yarborough appointed the panel and Benno Schmidt was asked to be its chairman. A Republican, he was an effective businessman and a good spokesman who did not pull his punches. He might have been unversed in science, but this was more than made up for by his organizational skills and his real sense of money. Dr. Krim's main responsibility would be to act as one of the voices for the scientists on the panel that Schmidt would chair, but this energetic, attractive figure also undertook to mobilize the scientists both for general support and for help in compiling that section of the report which would deal with the existing state of cancer research. She felt from the very beginning that at every stage of progress, from the report to the final bill, the panel must have a firm base in, and a good relationship with, the scientific community. This proved, however, to be a difficult task, and Dr. Krim needed all her powers of persuasion. One might think that the prospect of a concentrated attack on a difficult problem would be so attractive to the scientific community that they would be happy to help, for the appeal was very wide. Whether it was the prospect of more research money or a chance to contribute to the solution of a genuine human problem, there was something for scientists of all persuasions. Dr. Krim made many friends as the work progressed and was greatly helped by the warm active support from such scientific giants as Salvador Luria, Sol Spiegelman, James Watson, and Henry Kaplan, among others, but inevitably other people chose to see this effort only as an exercise in personal aggrandizement. It is also very hard to get scientists to take time out from their research to help with anything. So demonstrating either a traditional dislike of the political process or just sheer laziness, many scientists participated only reluctantly in the business.

They came forward with such reluctance that their later cries of pain about the deficiencies of the Cancer Act don't really evoke copious tears of sympathy. A number of consultants—Kingsley Sanders was one—came in to help Dr. Krim with the report. Two hundred scientists were ultimately contacted: getting them to answer letters, let alone detailed questions, was something of an agony.

The first meeting of Ralph Yarborough's panel took place in June, with further meetings held every week throughout the summer. At the end of August, Dr. Krim was ready to write the scientific part of the report, while the clinical sections were the responsibility of the specialists. Written in two and a half months flat, the joint effort of thirteen medical scientists and thirteen laymen, the final document is a remarkable piece of work. The section on the present state of cancer research is a most realistic statement which, with certain additions, could well stand as testimony today. After various specialists had testified before Ralph Yarborough's committee, the report was printed and issued on December 19.

In addition to Colonel Luke Quinn, another gun of the political activity was manned by Mike Gorman, another lobbyist to whom Mary Lasker had turned many times. They were both experienced and effective hands. They advised the panel on how to handle Senators and Congressmen, and mobilized support in favor of the bill. Perhaps much of their activity was superfluous, for to be against fighting cancer was to be against Mom, apple pie, and the flag. No one was going to begrudge the money or the effort, especially when compared with the Manhattan Project or the space race. If worthiness of the cause was the criterion, then support for cancer raised the political issue to the new level of idealism. When the rough conflicts came, they focused not on the question of whether, but how.

So by the fall of 1970, the pieces were more or less in place. The three most active people up to this point inevitably saw the problem in different terms. The pragmatic philanthropist had a somewhat simplistic view of the scientific difficulties; the financier conceived the fundamental problem as one of business management; the scientist had perhaps a naïve view of the capacity and willingness of her colleagues to spring into helpful action. But these differences were probably healthy, for everything progressed smoothly enough, and Yarborough's Subcommittee on Health heard evidence from many people who, like the initial panel of consultants before them, were most carefully chosen. They were all splendid witnesses.

Though one will never know the extent to which Yarborough thought that a public commitment to such an issue would help him attract votes, it is not really necessary to be cynical. For even before the fall of 1970 he had gone the way of Matthew Neely, having lost the democratic primary in the spring, to be replaced in the Senate, after the elections, by Lloyd Bentsen. Yarborough managed to produce a report by the end of 1970, however, and he had even introduced his Conquest of Cancer Bill into the Senate, though knowing it would die when the old Congress died. With any issue other than cancer, that might have been the end of it. A bill introduced is not a bill passed, and once one Congress is replaced by another, everything has to start all over again. This posed no real problem for Mary Lasker, however. She sprang back into action with new people. Edward Kennedy took over the chairmanship of the subcommittee, and Mary Lasker suggested that he now sponsor the bill. He was most happy to take the Yarborough Bill (S34) as it stood. He reintroduced it, and there were new hearings in the winter of 1971.

During the taking of testimony, Mrs. Anna Rosenberg Hoffman, a warm-hearted and energetic person, and a former Under Secretary of Defense, concentrated on the casualties of cancer, drawing attention to the great disparity between the numbers who died in Vietnam ("41,000 in six years") and those who died of cancer ("323,000 in one year"). The clinicians who gave evidence knew exactly what they wanted: not basic research so much as a new thrust towards cancer control and improved therapy. The scientists, too, knew what they wanted—money for basic research—and they pressed for it while keeping their feet firmly on the ground. No one ever held out the promise of a cure, no one ever held out the promise of total eradication, and analogies and comparisons with the moonshot were firmly discouraged. What was presented was a possibility only: that by a committed and high level of support, within the framework of a new and special agency independent of the National Institutes of Health, a real push forward could be made on the problem, a push which would lift our level of understanding, prevention and treatment to a new and more effective plane. But when things began to go wrong, as some things did, some of the fallout of cynicism and disillusionment inevitably spattered the scientific community. If the scientific statements as initially made were not exaggerated, but honest, why was this cynicism generated?

It is right to absolve the scientists—at this stage at least—of knowingly contributing to something which Lucy Eisenberg, writing in *Harper's* magazine (November 1971), characterized as, "the product of a high-powered P.R. campaign and a rather deceptive one at that." A few years later, Lee Edison would head an article in *Science Digest* with the title "The Cancer Rip-Off" (September 1974). In his syndicated column (January 23, 1974) Sidney J. Harris would say, "Cancer War is phony, just as I told you. I said it was a rotten, useless, wasteful, hysterical and emotional measure—just a cheap publicity stunt by the administration to make it look as if the U.S. were waging an 'all-out war' on cancer . . ." His language is almost worthy of Matthew Neely, but the new element in the equation is "the administration." Something went wrong on the way. What follows is an attempt to find out just what it was that went wrong. But note that like any account of a complicated historical situation—when seen and recorded from a distance by someone who was not intimately involved—this can only be a partial point of view.

To an extent, things had already begun to go awry in 1970. The seeds for future misunderstandings and conflicts were already sown, for the bill still lacked a committed endorsement by the scientific community. Perhaps time had been too short, but many subsequent problems might have been avoided if the report had been taken to various public and private agencies of the scientific community—the National Science Foundation, the National Academy, and the American Association for the Advancement of Science, for example—for their blessing on the project and the work of the consultants. There is such a thing as communal and institutional pride, and even given that scientists had not been wildly active initially, institutional approval of the idea and cooperation over strategy during the early stages might well have saved a lot of headaches later. Though this is certainly wisdom after the event the community could have united in an effort to counter the Nixon administration's politicizing of the issue.

For the foundations of the edifice, by then erected as a testament to a nation's commitment to the conquest of cancer, were now to be undermined by tunnels being dug towards it from two directions. The construction of both was predictable. On the one hand, the Nixon administration introduced a competing bill (S1828). The opportunity was too good to miss, especially when it involved stealing some thunder from a Kennedy. For Edward Kennedy and Senator Javits had reintroduced Yarborough's Conquest of Cancer Bill into the Senate on January 29, 1971. Eight days earlier, however, in his State of the Union address, President Nixon launched a biological moonshot, in language which held real promise. He stated:

> The time has come when the same kind of concentrated effort which split the atom and took Man to the Moon, should be turned towards conquering this dread disease . . . and—learning an important lesson from our space program—to organize those resources as effectively as possible.
>
> . . . Of all our research endeavors, cancer research may now be in the best position to benefit from a great infusion of sources. For there are moments in biomedical research when problems begin to break open and results begin to pour in, opening many new lines of inquiry and many new opportunities for breakthrough . . . We believe that cancer research has reached such a point.

The President asked for a hundred-million-dollar appropriation, a figure given to him by his long-time friend, Elmer Bobst, who for a number of years had a close and active association with the American Cancer Society. He had been chairman in the 1940's and was still a member of their board.

The level of public expectation was raised even higher by statements such as those from the weekly compilation of presidential documents, May 17, 1971.

> . . . The secretary of H.E.W. sent to the Congress today legislation that will set up a program, The Cancer Cure Program,

in the National Institutes of Health. This will differ from other programs in a very important respect.

. . . I have asked that it be independently budgeted and that it be directly responsible to the President of the United States . . . I believe that direct Presidential interest and Presidential guidance may hasten the day that we will find a cure for cancer. . . . *There have been some very significant breakthroughs, breakthroughs that indicated that we can really look forward to the day when we can find a cure for cancer.* [These italics are the President's, not mine.]

Though the whole tenor of the administration's statements was guaranteed to inspire confidence in the public sector, it did nothing for the confidence of the scientific community, who began to shoot down the man-on-the-moon analogy. Scientists pointed to the irrefutable fact that in cancer research we had nothing equivalent to the theoretical foundation that Newton provided for space travel, or Einstein provided for the atom bomb. We knew what we had to do in order to get to the moon: take a large lump of metal and light a big fire underneath it. But we still don't know what to do to cure cancer, because we still don't know what cancer really is.

If this was one point over which the scientists were unified, there was another that divided them. The real issue between Senator Kennedy's committee and the administration was the location of the new administrative structure. Who was going to be in charge of all that money? Who was going to implement the push toward the Conquest of Cancer? The panel had recommended a completely separate agency to deal with the conquest of cancer. The scientists were ambivalent about this, and they were acutely aware of the dangers which would arise if the whole program became politicized, directed by politicians and bureaucrats.

No one was against the Conquest of Cancer. The act was clearly going to pass, and the million letters that members of Congress later received in support of the National Cancer Act, from people mobilized by Ann Landers through her daily column, was one very crucial factor. But as someone said at the hearing, "They could . . . simply have presented the bill and it would have gone through the Senate." The one real issue that emerged from the testimony at the subcommittee hearings, during March and June 1971 was the issue of control and location. The panel felt that the situation demanded an expansion of cancer research at a rate which would simply not be possible within the system as it presently operated. For the bureaucratic barriers were too high to be surmounted quickly: there were too many points of critical decision-making, which inevitably increased the time lag between impulse and action. But the officials of HEW and NIH argued that the whole of biomedical research in America would suffer if cancer were hived off into an independent agency, and that since the problem of cancer was not comparable to putting a man on the moon, separating it out from general basic research in medicine and biology would fail to solve it. Moreover, they clearly resented the implication that bureaucratic attitudes and the tangle of red tape surrounding the people who work at NIH disqualified that institution from being an effective means for implementing a crash program. You might have needed a NASA for the moon, but you didn't need one for cancer. Not only was the timing inappropriate, for there was no theoretical matrix in which to imbed the effort, but an existing structure was already suitably geared for the administrative job.

These arguments, intensified by the probing questions of Senator Gaylord Nelson, who was consistantly opposed to an independent agency, made their mark; some scientists, such as Dr. Joshua Ledeberg, began backing away from their first position and finally supported a cancer agency within NIH, though others remained committed to the independent agency. What finally passed was the administration's bill, which was essentially identical with Yarborough's original document. There had been a hiatus at one point when nothing seemed to be moving, since two possible bills were floating around. Finally Benno Schmidt went to Senator Kennedy and asked if he would allow S84 to metamorphose into the administration's S1828. Kennedy agreed immediately, feeling that the issue was too important to be frustrated by political considerations. The bill had some elements of compromise, of course. The National Cancer Institute would remain within the framework of the National Institutes of Health, but with an independent budget which could be affected only directly by the President. In theory, the program was independent from both the NIH bureaucracy and the budget review, but the director of the cancer institute was still to report to the director of the National Institutes of Health. As for the President, he wanted his "cancer attack director" reporting to him alone, but he didn't get that either, for many people were of the same mind as Hubert Humphrey, who said in his testimony to the subcommittee: "I want to crack down on this business about reporting to the President. Now, most of that is sheer political theory and those of us who have been around here a little while, know it."

In one sense, the scientific community got hoisted with its own petard; in another sense a long-standing conflict was reapplied in a new setting. There is a profound suspicion of the "General Motors" approach to science, as if all that is needed is superb, efficient management. Conceivably, one could argue that where the theory and knowledge exist, the application of these depends on just those techniques of organization; if this had been so, all the panel had to do was recommend that Robert McNamara take over direction of the National Cancer Institute while society sat back and awaited results. It is highly questionable whether this approach works, however, and certainly it cannot work if it has nothing to work with. Though at that time there was a genuine difference of opinion among scientists as to whether or not a strong enough intellectual matrix existed to support an attack on a massive scale, everyone who testified in favor of the Cancer Act *had* to assume that it did. The only issue was whether the existing machinery would provide the best means, as the members of the HEW administration argued, or whether new organizations were necessary, as Benno Schmidt argued on behalf of his panel.

The expressed reservations of the scientists were compounded of old troubles. They were anxious to know how far back the chains of decision-making would stretch. They didn't mind that research should be coordinated, nor that a clearing house be set up to disseminate information about results, work and materials, but they were fearful of directed research. They were also very sensitive—wisely, as it turned out—to the issue of who was going to evaluate the worth of projects, and insisted that the system of external peer review, though not perfect, carried fewer dangers than contract research and internal evaluation within the framework of the NIH bureaucracy. At the same time they distrusted the flood tide of administrative propaganda, seeking to commit public resources to the program, since they felt the assessments were unrealistic, if not slightly devious. So it all added up: the possibility of government interference; the politicizing of research; the danger that a personally directed program, with an official who reported directly to the President, would mean that over the years NCI, then NIH and HEW, would do their best for Mr. Nixon rather than for the health of biomedical research in America.

Four years later we can see that, though much of the brouhaha was understandable, the dangers were much exaggerated. Research is going along well and generally the quality is good. But some things did not go right at all, and the widespread resentment that temporarily surfaced in 1973 and 1974 amongst the scientific and medical communities about the National Cancer Institute was only partly due to lack of institutional consultation earlier on. Other elements contributed to the resentment and at times bitterness.

The public relations approach was one. So far as this was concerned, there was a prophetic touch in an editorial in the April 21, 1971, issue of that most respected of all scientific journals, *Nature*. The author of the article, John Maddox, went straight to the heart of the matter. He pointed out that the combination of so much money, emotion and expectation and the precedent of the Manhattan Project had placed the American public in a position where it should reasonably expect a successful outcome as a result of this new national commitment. Though Maddox did not quote this, the following exchange between Representative Daniel Flood, a Democrat from Pennsylvania, and Carl Baker, the outgoing director of the National Cancer Institute, must be seen in the context of an endless stream of hopeful prognostication. It simply will not do to dismiss Flood's views as simplistic, though they may be. All he was doing was making a logical extrapolation from the utterances of those who stood, politically, to gain most from the war on cancer.

FLOOD: Every time the phone rings, I expect to pick it up and have you tell me that we have broken through in cancer virus (research).

BAKER: I don't think it happens as a breakthrough like that . . .

FLOOD: What day are you going to tell us, what month and year, "Here, Halleluja," as you have done with polio and measles?

BAKER: I don't think it is going to come that way.

What, John Maddox asked, would happen if those who took the money failed to deliver the goods, the goods that "public opinion has been led to expect"? Wouldn't the backlash be catastrophic, and could biological and medical research survive the disillusionment? There was also a Catch-22. If the cure did not arrive and the researchers who were now going to take such a hefty slice of the cancer cake later turned around and, to cover themselves, said that the time had not really been ripe for such a massive investment in cancer, wouldn't the disillusionment be total? Whatever happened, some recoil seemed inevitable, for the crusade for a cancer cure was acquiring the same quality as the crusade against polio. Nothing less than an equally successful outcome would be tolerated. Consequently, the article argued, the state of the art was such that the best procedure for the new czar—whoever was appointed to head the National Cancer Institute—would be to hedge his bets and concentrate on basic research. You can't go far wrong with knowledge.

In his testimony on March 20 before the Subcommittee on Public Health and Environment of the Committee on Interstate and Foreign Commerce (House of Representatives), Dr. James Watson put this problem in his typically colorful language. He admitted his bias from the very beginning, for his job as director of the Cold Spring Harbor Laboratories places him in charge of a major research program on viruses and cancer. His statement was a realistic assessment of the state of the art. It was also a personal testimony of a widely shared faith about just what it takes to guarantee progress in a branch of science. As Watson saw it, the lines of disagreement between the scientific community and the administration were drawn up between a group who promised a degree of success in the cancer crusade, provided the scientific game was played according to long-tried rules, and an administration with a philosophical commitment to the American ethic of self-help. They would pay for achievement, not promise. But if promise was not yet obvious, then some all-encompassing slogan could be utilized as a temporary stopgap, to satisfy society's expectations for the time being. The plan supplanted the problem, and the message was supplanting the action.

> By careful public relations the impression can be created that we are onto something hot . . . The fact that many of us think that viruses are the cause of cancers can be construed that an effective vaccine is just around the corner, maybe by the time of the 1976 Bi-centennial. But this is awful hogwash! . . . We are told that immunological tricks are almost worked out . . . but here again such claims are not based on a thorough understanding of the basic biology, which still does not exist, but more in the hopes that if we say immunology, often enough, cancer cells will just give up and die . . . Current reports to the National Cancer Board about the future of current chemotherapeutic approaches invariably remind me of Pentagon briefings where the courteous, upright colonels know that they will never gain their stars if the two-star generals get the impression that the battle will not soon be won . . . I see no rational alternative to many more years of firm support to the better of our scientists who work on the problems that either directly or indirectly bear on cancer . . .

Watson did not exaggerate the public relations "sell," which is still believed to be essential in order to bring in the money. But this "sell" also brings in a whole battery of pressures on the scientists, who become resentful in their turn. For what does it take to get support? The answer is, apparently, expectation and promise. But what should it take? The answer is realism and truth. This may be gross political naïveté on my part, but naïveté may be no worse than cynicism. Eventually the public may see through the sell, and may also realize that science administrators and public affairs officers are following a line to which in their hearts they may not subscribe. This will breed cynicism on both sides, and in science, just as in politics, an atmosphere of cynicism or mistrust is the worst possible one in which to conduct our affairs.

The mistrust can be internal, too; sometimes there are resentments amongst those who work the other arm of cancer: the doctors. The cancer clinician who told me, "White man at NIH, he speak with forked tongue," was moved to this remark over his own experience with a news release by NIH that B.C.G. vaccine had effected a cure in cancer. "To use the term 'cure' for

B.C.G. at this stage was very upsetting," he said, "for B.C.G. is not terribly well understood in terms of what it does, or did even in that one case. The theoretical aspects of stimulating the immune system are not understood."

But the episode resulted in the relatives of his tumor patients calling from Miami, from Seattle, from all over the country, saying, "Why isn't Aunt Millie getting B.C.G.; why aren't you treating her right?" "So I called one of the persons—one of the administrators at the NCI," he told me, "who relates with the physicians there, and asked him if he was aware that the press articles on B.C.G. had caused a lot of reaction. He said yes, he'd had lots of telephone calls, too. So I also asked him if he was aware of the anxieties he was causing on the part of the patients and families; they were anxious that they should be getting the most up-to-date, and judging from the press release, the most potent treatment? He said no, he really wasn't aware of this. So then I said, now that you have released this information, could you please give me some B.C.G. to use? I live in Cumberland, Maryland, which is on top of the mountains not too far from you, and I am also a licensed clinical drug investigator, in oncology. The answer came back over the phone, 'Well, this is a Phase Three drug, and only two or three people in the country have permission to use it.' So I said to him, 'Why in hell didn't you see that the article said that? Why weren't you as meticulous in the process of issuing this information as you are in advertising it? You knew very well what it was going to do.' "

They had a very bruising conversation. I asked him, "How did the NCI official answer your direct question, 'Why in hell didn't you see that the article said that?' " My friend replied, "He said, 'These things happen': a bureaucratic answer which gives you no satisfaction at all. But then I didn't expect to have any satisfaction other than venting my spleen; that was my psychotherapy for the morning. On the one hand, the people at the NCI have a tendency to be very haughty to those of us outside, and they are not scrupulously fair on the other. They don't even have to exaggerate; they simply drop out anything that is negative. They don't claim universal cure; they simply extrapolate. From saying two cases of melanoma have been cured, they drop the 'two' and say 'cases,' and so it goes on. It's not right."

A second source of friction relates to bureaucracy. This has its own particular variations of Parkinson's Law, not only expanding to fill up all available space and absorb all available money, but also, once having been brought into existence, proceeding to create conditions that justify and insure that existence. One of my medical colleagues has propounded Swisher's First Law of Cancer Research, which reads, "Ultimately all cancer-related activities become malignant themselves." Certain activities of all bureaucratic institutions may well be directed as much to self-perpetuation as anything else.

A further problem was the politicizing of the National Institutes of Health. The question came down to one of allegiance. Where was the final allegiance of this organization? Was it to biomedical research or to the political administration? A decade ago this question would have been quite outrageous, for there was no doubt. But in the past few years the pendulum has swung in the other direction as administrators rushed to demonstrate their control and accountability in times of tight money. The emphasis was on specific research targets, and this resulted in certain areas receiving much more money than others. The need to account to the government managers in HEW meant that political considerations rather than scientific ones sometimes determined policy and the overall attitudes of NIH personnel.

Some of the problems were in the area of contract research. Though funds were still given by the grant system—in which anyone who had a worthwhile scientific project would apply to NIH for money and the project would be assessed by a committee of peers—a significant proportion of the money came through the contract research system. Under this system, however, the in-house scientists and administrators of NIH formulate the framework for research, identifying the areas that should be studied and searching for people to do the job. The contracts are given for a specific scientific task, cover a limited time span, and are reviewed every year. Some of them are passed on to semiscientific industrial concerns as well as to members of the scientific community. On the face of it, the system does have the merit of focusing scientific effort and also providing a means whereby scientists are consistently accountable for their activities, and therefore for the money, to the people who act on society's behalf. The aspect of accountability is perfectly proper, in my opinion, but other aspects of contract research have led to what one scientist described to me as the "death of science" in this country.

There are several snags. One is that, until quite recently, it has been the in-house scientists of NCI, that new breed of science administrators, who have formulated the frameworks for obtaining the contracts. One temptation is obvious—namely, to open opportunity in their own particular special field. Though the quality of work is partly judged from outside, the opinions of the inside scientists carry the greatest weight. It is difficult to fight those who are generating the momentum within the existing framework, so the NIH people are almost judge and jury both of what should be done and whether it was being done well.

Another piquant aspect of contract research has been the tendency to apply for money for projects the results of which are already known. Some scientists insist that this is inevitable in the present system. The main criterion for an award is the capacity to demonstrate the relevance of the project to the program's target. But the only sure way to prove this relevance is to have, in fact, already proved it. This is never admitted in one's contract proposal, of course, though everyone is aware of what is happening. While the application is written in the future tense, the work may well already be in the past.

Contracts also show other incestuous tendencies. Dr. Anfinsen, who received a Nobel Prize for Chemistry in 1973, once asked a very simple question at a National Cancer Institute meeting: just how do contracts originate? He was told that the ideas are mostly put forward by the investigators themselves at the annual meeting for contractors. Even though NCI sometimes did get a good, unsolicited proposal, they still had to see whether or not it fitted in with the general program. But how could one know, Anfinsen asked, whether they were missing something important? How can such contracted research exploit the surprises, the unexpected, the possibility, as in the platinum story, that someone from a way-out field might have something vitally important to contribute?

Criticism of the National Cancer Institute and this system reached its apogee recently when a special committee appointed by the National Cancer Board headed by Dr. Norton Zinder was called in to review the activity of the Special Virus Cancer Program, S.V.C.P. The scenario and end result of S.V.C.P. had also been predicted by John Maddox. Pointing out that Congress and the administration were already vying with each other over "just how to organize the spending spree," Maddox had highlighted this danger: that tides of enthusiasm and fashion, such as those that swept along research on RNA tumor viruses, would produce a situation in which cancer research would become a synonym for a study of a few potentially exciting and fashionable interests, to the exclusion of much else. The in-house people both chose the work and assessed it. As it happened, 10 percent of the NCI budget ended up in the S.V.C.P., directed by a group of people in a manner designed to gladden the hearts of the NCI administrators. The program was right on target and directed with an overall aim clearly in mind: the relationship between RNA viruses and human cancer. But there was an exaggerated emphasis on this particular facet. In one of the understatements of the year, the Zinder report on the program said that "if the first definitive human cancer virus turns out to be one of the many suspect DNA viruses (rather than an RNA virus), the S.V.C.P. would be in a strange position." So inevitably, as James Watson has said, "Bad feelings about the S.V.C.P. exist because there are a lot of virologists who share the same goals. The ones in S.V.C.P. are very rich. The others, who are just as good, were just poor."

The activities fitted most beautifully into the NCI's overall scheme. The three chairmen of the three large segments, Drs. Heubner, Todaro, and Manaker, dispensed nine million dollars, seven million dollars and twelve million dollars per year respectively. The contracts for research within their areas were awarded by a working group appointed by these segment chairmen, who tended to name to these groups the very people receiving the contracts. The spiral turned in on itself. Two of the segment chairmen were also branch chiefs, controlling contract money and large research programs within NCI by virtue of their position as segment heads. Not only that, but these people were project officers, too—that is, they were committed to oversee the day-to-day operations of the contracts. In this way they controlled or supervised the work of operations amounting to some ten million dollars a year, one-fourth of the

total program. The Zinder report, in another classic understate-
ment, said, "There is an inordinate amount of power in the
segment chairman's group . . . which accounts for the antipathy
for the program in the scientific community."

The questions piled up. Was there sufficient intellectual
justification for concentrating this amount of money on RNA
viruses in the first place? Should outside advice and the usual
system of checks and balances which govern other research
programs have been dispensed with here? Does a hectic pace in a
mass attack speed solutions? For a 1971 article in *Science*,
Nicholas Wade interviewed many virologists, who said such
things as: there were "possibilities of incredible fiascos"; one
could "delete most of the work financed under contract to
S.V.C.P. and we would be almost as far along the road as we are
now"; "The bulk of the program is still really a bunch of
worthless junk, such as injecting monkeys with God knows
what." S.V.C.P. had begun to acquire the same reputation as
the chemotherapy program did in earlier years when it was
known in the trade as the nothing-too-stupid-to-test program. It
must be emphasized, however, that the integrity of the people
concerned was never in question. They were just doing what
they had been asked to do, and were in no way flimflamming the
public. The system had just evolved in such a way that there was
no direct accountability to peer groups.

Moreover, it must also be pointed out however that it is
unfair to lay the onus for any deficiencies in the implementation
of the National Cancer Act solely on the shoulders of people
within NCI. The fact remains that many outside scientists called
in to review projects simply do not bother to do their
homework. If they fail to read proposals really carefully they will
also fail to ask the hard question, to mount the tough
intellectual challenge. It is the meeting of this challenge alone
which will demonstrate whether the project in question is good
or merely mundane. But too often this task has been left to the
poor, hard-working administrator. In any case, some of the
defects highlighted by the Zinder report have been rectified. In
the spring of 1974 it was decided that the review committees for
contract research should be composed totally of outside scientists.

The system with its pattern of activity emerged naturally from the context of an overall master plan. A National Cancer Panel, a trinity of one layman and two scientists set up to monitor the bureaucracy, was quickly created and planning sessions inaugurated. But Dr. James Watson felt that the massive three-volume *National Cancer Plan*, a production aided by a public relations firm for the not inconsiderable sum of one million dollars, served to obscure the real nature of the cancer problem even further.

The provisions of the National Cancer Act of 1971 laid down that the director of the National Cancer Institute had to put forward a five-year plan which would be updated every year. Consequently, a series of meetings of NCI administrators and 250 cancer specialists took place between October 1971 and March 1972 in Arlie House, Virginia. James Watson called them "soporific orgies." The basic outline of the Plan had already been drawn up by a former NCI Director, Carl Baker, and Louis Carrese, a systems-management specialist. Initially, Dr. Carl Baker had planned to run things his own way, but he had been stung by criticism that his ideas were too clinically orientated. So he called these sessions to allow scientists and administrators to have a "shot" at planning the action. But after he had left the institute, one legacy was a Plan which few people really understood and which quickly came to resemble an engulfing monster. Partly by a simple exercise, during which every one of the specialists wrote down every single way they could think of to approach cancer research, a totally comprehensive catalogue was finally produced: one might call it *A Guide for Aspiring Patrons.* According to Carrese, it was to be "meaningful" to everybody. The single goal of reducing cancer morbidity in all its aspects fanned out into seven objectives, which in turn fanned out into a series of approaches. These divided yet again into a set of "approach elements," and finally, into the threads of ultimate refinement, a list of "project areas," the point where the research is actually done. It can, of course, be put in pictorial terms. So a diagram of a wheel, a visual analogue of the objectives and approaches implicit in the total cancer program, hangs on the wall of many laboratories and offices throughout the National Institutes of Health. But as Barbara Culliton, a staff writer of *Science*, pointed out, the diagram can either be taken quite seriously or be interpreted as Pop Art, depending upon whose wall it is on.

Approaches like this are totally foreign to the scientific community. This of itself does *not* necessarily mean that they are irrelevant or mistaken, but one must, for the moment, look at the rationale which underlies the whole approach. Science has done some remarkable things in the course of its history, and the question is this: is a concerted approach based on this kind of systems planning and management going to enable scientists to do science better and faster? If it isn't, then the whole exercise is a waste of time as well as a costly exercise. Part of the difficulty is that we shall, of course, never know the truth. If the cancer problem is effectively solved in five years, which I very much doubt can happen, then nearly everyone will point to this massive directed effort as the prime reason for success. But if, as seems much more likely, the whole problem takes a couple of decades, then we may never be sure. The question is an important one: is money a necessary *and* a sufficient condition both for the growth of science and for an increase in the rate of scientific discovery? Undoubtedly money is necessary, but something over and above the money has to be added. Here one finds, in its essentials, the crucial differences between administrators on the one hand, and the scientific community on the other. The administrators believe that over and above the scientist's daily research, the "extra" is planning, organization, management, identification of research areas, and direction toward that work deemed necessary for an attack on the disease. The research, therefore, becomes centralized, and herein lies the rub.

The present rationale behind the cancer plan reveals one fundamental assumption: there can be an overall plan for discoveries in science even where what is involved is fundamental theory rather than technological application. It assumes that money can guarantee, if not everything, at least something. But even though you *can* pay for brains, can you also buy ideas? Most scientists would go along with Peter Medawar, who said, "Ideas are the life blood of science. They can't be bought, they can sometimes be sold." Perhaps the most one can hope for is to assemble the best pool of minds, give them the right kind of conditions . . . and pray.

While saying this, we have to admit that our understanding of those conditions that guarantee good scientific work, and ergo scientific discoveries, is lamentable. If we did know, we *might* be able to come up with and apply a reasonable managerial policy for science. We all have our own personal ideas on the subject. I doubt that history tells us all that much, either, since one of the fascinating things is to see the enormous variety of people and situations that have brought good science forward. The nature of scientific creativity remains one of science's most elusive mysteries. But scientists are in accord on what you can't do—namely, order on demand, especially if the problem itself is extremely diverse. You have to spread your net widely, though this does not mean spreading your largesse thinly. If one can identify—as one can—both those broad areas where the problem is likely to give and those obviously fundamental to our understanding of malignant transformations, then one can hope eventually to lift our level of understanding and therapeutic application to a higher plane.

In a field where such an enormous degree of creative imagination is necessary, imaginative flexibility is perhaps even more important than management. Though the administrators at NCI swear that one of the joys of the Plan is the very flexibility it allows, scientists are not so sure, for when you are working on a contract, you are not permitted to deviate. Yet so much of scientific experience shows that from one question, new ideas and possibilities emerge, springing out sometimes from the oddest and most unlikely places. These possibilities may be immensely valuable to follow for their own sake, but they may also have important and as yet unknown consequences. I saw this happen over and over again during my time at the Sloan-Kettering Institute. One day Alf Burness said to me that one of the most stultifying things about filling out an application—even for a grant, let alone a contract—was that it in no way reflected the process of discovery. He said, "I would like to say, 'and at this point I confidently expect to make a mistake. But this mistake will generate a new idea that must be explored because it might be fruitful.' " But he certainly wouldn't be able to go on in this fashion under the contract system, for one had to stay dead on target. These rigid frameworks and confining schemes have a stifling effect which many scientists dislike thoroughly.

Another implicit assumption highlights the most fundamental weakness of the whole Plan: namely, that there is a pattern in creativity, which can not only be discerned, but actually exploited. This is quite wrong. Patterns of creativity are basically very variable. In one situation, a loner can do something that is very significant; in another there has to be a team. One wonders whether variety and diversity both in people and effort really can be planned for. The failure to appreciate the patterns of creativity is the great weakness of modern scientific administration. We now have a large professional corps of science administrators who know that it is much easier to deal with standardized people and standardized approaches than with irritating geniuses. There is no consistent pattern at all in genius, and this fact too *is* irritating, but genius is what we may need.

The final gripe added to all this was perhaps the most serious of all, a factor contributing to a general malaise, though now the blame cannot be laid at the door of NIH. Compared with other branches of biomedical research, the National Cancer Institute has been forging ahead. It has done so at a time when severe financial cutbacks have occurred in almost every other area, and most critically in the training of pre- and postdoctoral scientists. This budgetary decision of the Nixon administration threatened to neutralize the program with horrible effectiveness. The strength of the enterprise depends on the quality of people coming up from below who can challenge existing patterns of thought. The fatal disease of scientific old age, with no known cure, is hardening of the categories. But there is an antidote to the disease, and this takes the form of challenging young Turks. Dr. James Watson made this explicit in an article in the February 26, 1972, issue of the *New Republic*. He raised the question of who should get "all that new money." He had no doubt at all; he felt it should go to younger people, via the creation of a number of institutes like McArdle Laboratory at Wisconsin, where small groups of some ten independent investigators work, each with a problem that focused on some aspect of molecular biology relating to cancer. But, Watson argued, such is the gerontocracy in science that the young men with the brilliant ideas, the generation from which one expects the imaginative insights, were far more likely to be found sitting stuck to the laboratory bench while their elders grabbed the opportunity and the cash. Or, as Watson put it, "The current superstars on the cancer scene would be getting even more money to bolster their egos." But the real target of his fire was the way the science training program had been allowed to slacken seriously. This slack continued for a while, but in 1973, money was finally released for predoctoral and postdoctoral training. The initial commitment was for two years only, however: a constant underpinning of the training program will be necessary for much longer.

That is what went wrong with the system, but we must also ask: what is going right? Actually, plenty is right. Though many of the caveats are justified, some of the dangers have been grossly exaggerated. Possibly the most important consequence of the program is the public enthusiasm that has been generated. Though the second Law of Cancer Research states, "The degree of real progress is inversely proportional to the number of announced breakthroughs," the public is aware that real progress is being made, though they are sometimes misled as to its speed and extent. From all the work, and from the recent public knowledge and optimism that attended such episodes as Betty Ford's and Happy Rockefeller's operations, we see that cancer is a problem that clearly can be handled. If any reservations must remain, they do so, as Sir Alexander Haddow pointed out, because of its "high inherent recalcitrance." The inference we should draw from all this, as I see it, is that if massive support for research is to be effective, there must be a *continuing commitment*, for an atmosphere of continuous justification is destructive, both to the scientists and to the speedy solution of the problem. All disciplines prosper best in a steady-state atmosphere; a highly political situation, with budget cuts producing a series of uncertain oscillations, is bound to halt the momentum.

We have seen that one problem of federal funding is an inherent conservatism which in the end is self-defeating. The control of funding tends to be concentrated in the hands of one ingroup, and this continues until another ingroup takes over. The danger is that conventional work, work which is in line with the prevailing scientific dogma, gets higher priority and is funded at the expense of the rest.

So independent funding from external sources with both prestige and power, such as the American Cancer Society and private foundations, is an essential and valuable counterforce whereby unconventional and broad speculation can be given their outlet and in areas other than pure research private sources have played a pivotal role. The American Cancer Society has again been crucial here. Their level of research support has already been mentioned, but they promote three other equally vital types of activity. The society plays a valuable educational role in the area of public information; it supports therapeutic and clinical work; and it can call on some two and a half million volunteers whose activities cover the spectrum from fund-raising to chauffeuring patients to treatment centers, to assistance in the recovery programs designed especially to help those patients who have had severely disabling operations. The main problem the American Cancer Society faces is that of raising money, for all its funds are privately donated, and a large proportion of the effort of its "private army" is concentrated on this job. One must recognize that once again the appeal has to touch those responsive chords in the public, chords of emotion and promise. But the American Cancer Society has always been both honest and thoroughly realistic in its appeal.

The role of the private institutions, therefore, is very important. Bob Good sees it as crucial, not only because of the money, but because it reflects society's commitment to the program. However, society should understand thoroughly just what this commitment entails. Bob said, "If we turn this over totally to the government, it means we as a culture are not willing to engage directly in this search." I am not certain about the validity of his argument, since in a democracy the commitments of the government are supposed to reflect the commitments of the people. But I think what was in his mind was an issue to which Americans remain highly sensitive. Which is best, direct self-help or centralized decisions made at a distance? The problem of financing cancer research puts this issue in a very simple perspective. Since the early twenties, ever since the U.S. government began to support cancer research and Congress voted fifty thousand dollars in response to Matthew Neely's plea, the aggregate amount for all of the Conquest of Cancer programs has amounted to just what it took to put one big space lab into the air. This is a tremendous amount of money, but Bob Good feels it still isn't going to be enough to do a major job in science. It would not have put a man on the moon, nor could it have solved any other major program.

Yet money alone really isn't the only issue: the commitment of people is, and this is where the self-help comes in. This means being willing to act as helpers in many ways, of which private finance is only one. The critical necessity is to keep the cutting edge of research fine and sharp, and one way to do this is to present counterbalancing forces to the huge resources of the National Institutes of Health. Independent institutions such as Sloan-Kettering, the university departments in America and Europe, and the Imperial Cancer Research Fund in London— all in their own ways combine to provide these forces.

At the level of the individual scientist, the program is going well for other reasons. Kingsley gave me one small example of a scientist's new satisfactions. "At the end of every experimental program, there always are one or two small, niggling loose ends that prevent you settling down into a state of comfortable certainty, and inhibit the peace of mind that comes when a problem has been parcelled up. When funds are as generous as they now are, these loose ends can be tied up rapidly. It is much more satisfactory." Tom Connors in England gave me another example. We were speaking about the program at NIH of screening possible anticancer compounds. He pointed out that those of us outside were rather too smug. NIH did all the technical work, and the rest of us felt able to criticize it because it got nowhere. Tom himself felt that not only was this screening something that *had* to be done but also a second service was being provided to the rest of the world—namely, a facility where the compounds people discovered can be tested as rapidly as possible. He and other scientists can get answers on a compound or on a patient from NIH within a year. This is very rapid; and no other facility on the same scale exists anywhere else.

The Plan is also going "right" for other reasons. The sheer amount of basic research that is done will affect many other fields besides cancer. It already has: one has only to remember the links that foetal antigens provide between transplantation surgery and cancer to realize that the ripples which flow out are going to have an important effect in many branches of medicine.

The relative roles of other, much poorer countries in the field can sometimes be a sensitive issue, but amongst the international community I found a sense of the realities of life, rather than jealousy. Admittedly I have heard some people in Europe reacting sourly to the lavish spending, with the "comforting" convictions that money can only take you a little way. They are matched by people in America, mostly from the Public Information Departments, who equally sourly reported that, "The rest of the world is content to leave it to us." But most views on this matter, such as Tom Connors', were balanced and generous. Avrion Mitchison, for instance, sees the differences between the approaches of American and British science as only ones of degree. European science is just smaller, but in proportion Europeans do their share. Medical science is mostly American, and what isn't done there, while it can be of very good quality and contribute greatly to the advancement of learning, is almost a side show but *only* because that work would have been done in America before long. Americans may be richer, they may have more scientists at work, and this quantitative difference may be reflected in the proportion of discoveries. What is far more interesting are the special ways in which the Americans are cleverer than the Europeans and the special ways Europeans are cleverer than Americans. Americans do have much greater intellectual mobility: one sees this in all disciplines, not just science. Students are brought up to move much more agilely; they become set along intellectual lines much later, if at all. They are tremendously constructive, though not always reflective. The American figure that Avrion respects highly is the prototype engineer, who looks at a problem and is concerned not with what is true or false, not with who said what first or what this is going to do to his career, but with identifying the real problem and finding the solution. In science, as in other fields, they are extreme pragmatists.

On the other hand, the spirit of competitiveness evokes great and damaging suspicion. In Europe senior scientists can be found happily collaborating together; you also find these same men in the laboratory. American scientists tend to get driven out into administration or entrepreneurship in middle age, so when an English scientist asked me how many people amongst the emperors of the cancer institutes I actually found up to their elbows in blood or tissue culture, I had to admit it was a fair question. In the frenetic atmosphere Americans pay lip service to serendipity but seldom give themselves enough time to allow it to work. Like so many other things in America, science too is larger than life. The results and the money are quantitatively greater than anywhere else. The number of personnel and sheer size of the operation is sometimes quite overwhelming. So, too, are those unquantifiable aspects of science which at times provide distortions and an unhealthy competition.

Thus, if one concludes that in certain respects, patronage of cancer research in the United States carries elements of both encumbrance and blessing, this comes not from the initial intention, which was generous and right, but from a number of extraneous factors foreign to science as it is traditionally practiced. Competition may be good; it may, as Bob Good insists, "continually sharpen the cutting edge," but I suspect it has now reached such a degree in American science that it brings unwelcome pressure on everyone, on scientists, on society and on those who inhabit the buffer state between. If society really understood the nature of the cancer problem, which it was not allowed to, then it could take an adult view of its contract. As a society we should have been told, by politicians as well as by scientists, that science can not be very precise about when our understanding of cancer will come, nor about the rate in which cures will follow. But at least we know enough to be optimistic about progress, and we also have the parameters to make a mature judgment about the commitment, both with regard to time scale and money. The young people we should be training so as to maintain a long-term program will require support at yet another level, for though money can be turned on and off like a tap, discoveries cannot. Making discoveries is not like making profits, and to demand the same measure of guarantees as exists in business is to hold a sword of Damocles over the heads of people who should be free to get on with the task we have set them. The real problem is how to involve the best scientific minds in cancer research, not "managing" them once they are there.

So I find it piquant that, five years after she had received the phone call from Mrs. Mary Lasker, Dr. Mathilde Krim could tell me, albeit with a charming smile, "We didn't really need the Plan; all we needed was the money."

7

CANCER AND SCIENTISTS:
THE GOD WITHIN MAN

Hadn't I always known that science and philosophy elaborate them-
selves, in spite of all the passions and narrowness of men, in spite of the
vanities and weaknesses of their servants, in spite of all the heated
disorder of contemporary things? Wasn't it my own phrase to speak of,
'That greater mind' in men, in which we are but moments and
transitorily-lit cells?

—Remington (*The New Machiavelli*,
by H. G. Wells)

IF SCIENTISTS have intellectual fidgets about the world, then I
have intellectual fidgets about scientists. I could never entirely
separate the ideas I was trying to understand from the men who
were creating them. Not that I tried particularly hard, since the
interplay between the two is always intriguing. Scientists are not
all alike, and they bring to their study of nature as much variety
as nature presents to them. They are unselfish enough to say
that they will play the game of scientific discovery by a particular
set of rules, but that said, the rest is frankly quite personal.

If objectivity is present in science so, too, is immense
subjectivity. What you do and how you do it may be circum-
scribed by the rules of the game, but within those rules you can
play according to your own strategy and manner, national style
even, as did all the scientists I met. The French approach to
science has an air of clear Cartesian logic, a devotion to rational
thought and pure ideas, as if they wished to operate on a higher

mental plane, certainly when compared with the earthier quality of their English counterparts. Lord Kelvin is reported to have said often, "If ye kin make a model, ye understand it; if you canna, ye dinna." So full of models was his laboratory that Pierre Duhem, the famous French physicist, was thunderstruck when he first saw the paraphernalia that adorned Kelvin's room: pulleys, wires, clanking machinery. He was moved to utter with, I am sure, that look of baffled resignation wherewith most Frenchmen contemplate all things English, "We thought we were entering the tranquil abode of reason, and lo, we find ourselves in a factory." There was also a simple, but in its time famous, experiment in which a scientist took a fertilized frog's egg and set one half of it in a current of warm water, and the other half in a current of cold water. He wanted to see whether the temperature influenced the development of the egg in any way, but, as Paul Weiss remarked to me, "Only a man who has spent half of his life in front of a fire, with his backside burning and his front freezing, could have thought this experiment up. It had to be an Englishman." It was.

While one must resist making too many generalizations about national character and national scientific styles, the differences are nevertheless very real. It is obvious, even to the outsider, not only that the scale of British research is small compared to America's, but that being poor is now an accepted part of the British way of science, though I question whether the austerity need be carried quite so far. Many of the American laboratories were equally small, equally crammed, but in England, I missed the cartoons, the pictures, the music, the irreverent and irrelevant impedimenta. Peter Alexander's office was the only one that was quite lively. Everyone assured me that it is all due to the essential streak of Puritanism in the English character, carried over in the form of puritanical science. I am not convinced, for I think Americans have far more of that quality. But puritanical or not, there *is* a whiff of Sir Francis Drake in the British, a "We have time for this game of bowls before we beat the Spaniards"—a languid attitude but one which sometimes pays great dividends. There is a deceptive air in English science which an American friend was gently blaspheming several years back. He was to share the Nobel Prize with an English colleague whose leisurely work and progress were haunting him at that time. The quality of measured deliberation wafting across the Atlantic was maddening; it was, as he said, "blowing his mind." Yet these two men scaled the Olympian heights of science together. How little of any of this has ever come out.

For generations our image of the scientist was a myth—and partly a self-sustaining one. This was clearly shown nearly twenty years ago when Margaret Mead and Rhoda Métraux published the results of a pilot study on the image of a scientist among high school students of America—a study undertaken at a time when there was an urgent call for more scientists.* Future scientists would have to emerge from this group if they emerged at all. The study reflected the students' attitudes toward science as a result of their contacts through teaching or the media. One of their images was a very positive one: science as an activity which greatly benefited society through its contributions to health, defense, and life in general. This stood in marked contrast to a second, negative image: the human one that emerged when the questions shifted to their personal choices.

I took the composite human portraits in their paper, originally published in *Science*, and set it against the personal equivalents of the people I had come to know so well.

"The scientist is a man who wears a white coat and works in a laboratory. He is elderly or middle-aged and wears glasses." . . . "The sparkling white laboratory is full of sounds; the bubble of liquids in test tubes and flasks, the squeaks and squeals of laboratory animals, the muttering voice of the scientist." . . . "He experiments with plants and animals, cutting them apart, injecting serum into animals . . . He writes neatly in black books."

This fitted quite well, except that none of my scientists, young or old, wrote neatly.

"He is a very intelligent man—a genius or almost a genius. He is interested in his work and takes it seriously. He is careful, patient, devoted, courageous, open-minded. He works for long hours in the laboratory, sometimes day and night, going without food or sleep. He wants to know the answer. One day he may straighten up and shout; 'I've found it! I've found it.' The scientist is a truly

* "Image of the Scientist Among High-School Students: A Pilot Study," *Science* 126, no. 3270 (1957): 384–390.

wonderful man. Where would we be without him? The future rests on his shoulders."

The divergence was beginning.

"The scientist is a brain. His work is uninteresting, dull, monotonous, tedious, time-consuming." . . . "If he works by himself, he is alone and has heavy expenses. If he works for a big company, he has to do as he is told. . . . He is just a cog in a machine." . . . "He may not believe in God or lose his religion. His belief that Man is descended from animals is disgusting. He is a brain; he is so involved in his work that he doesn't know what is going on in the world. He has no other interests and neglects his body for his mind. He can only talk, eat, breathe and sleep science."

"He neglects his family—pays no attention to his wife, never plays with his children. He has no social life, no other intellectual interests, no hobbies or relaxations. He bores his wife, his children and their friends—for he has no friends of his own or knows only other scientists—with incessant talk which nobody else can understand; he is never home. He brings home work and also bugs and creepy things. He is always running off to his laboratory. . . . A scientist should not marry. No one wants to be a scientist or wants to marry one."

Running through these composite portraits are, of course, certain threads of accuracy, but of all the conclusions in this study, I think one is most important. The students had never realized that there was, or could be, sheer delight in the intellectual activity, that it could be rewarding in itself. It may be an expression of the way it was presented to them at school, but there was a deadness about the enterprise. Science didn't come alive; it was populated either by ghosts or dead men. It is as if they were presented with a heap of stones, and were told from that alone to imagine a city of living, breathing people. Perhaps we in society cannot be entirely to blame for these misconceptions, for people who ought to have known better perpetuated the myth. In one of his last novels, *Meantime*, H. G. Wells wrote:

"The disease of cancer will be banished from life by calm, unhurrying, persistent men and women, working, with every shiver of feeling controlled and suppressed, in hospitals and laboratories. And the motive that will conquer cancer will not be pity nor horror; it will be the curiosity to know how and why."

"And the desire for service," said Lord Tamar.

"As the justification of that curiosity," said Mr. Sempack, "but not as the motive. Pity never made a good doctor; love never made a good poet. Desire for service never made a discovery."

I remember my small surge of anger when I first read that, an emotion which the passage consistently triggers. To be as charitable to Wells as I can, he was perhaps arguing only that an overwhelming emotional desire to cure cancer must not be allowed to get in the way of a critical assessment of the present state of knowledge. Scientists do not, should not, indulge in wishful thinking, but when I thought of Stuart, Janez and Jim, I could see that so often their motives, *as well* as their justifications, were compounded of pity, desire for service and sometimes sheer human concern—which is another name for love. Wells was cold, cold and wrong; in these words he drained this human endeavor of its human content. Of course, the desire for service alone will never make a good scientist, no more than would pity alone. To these qualities, and to the natural quivering curiosity, must be added scientific judgment, knowledge of scientific techniques and the strategies. The Dr. Strangelove image that Wells draws for us here is the image that has persisted, but it bears as little relation to the reality as do the distorting mirrors in a seaside amusement park.

But what is it that really distinguishes scientists both from us and from each other, and how do their differences affect the science they create? The traits that set them apart from the rest of us were admirably caught by Gip Wells in the aphorism that described Kingsley so aptly. Those intellectual fidgets, the mental restlessness, the love of enigmas poured forth from all the scientists I met and had probably been a feature of their personalities from the very beginning. I remember one week when I was constantly riding the Sloan-Kettering wagon, and riding with me each day was the same quiet young man who spent the entire journey with his head buried in scientific articles. He never uttered a word, never responded to Bernie's teasing or to the amusing reflections of Bill Martin, the senior driver. I thought that this shy, fair-haired fellow must be studying for his preliminary exams, for I had never seen such quiet obsession. But one day we bumped into each other in the hall, and I learned that he was still only a schoolboy.

Scott Freeman was seventeen years old and worked at the Sloan-Kettering Institute laboratories as a volunteer in his free time. He had stayed much longer than the usual one summer vacation; in fact, he came in whenever he could. His enthusiasm had been most munificently rewarded, for he had been granted a long and encouraging interview with Lloyd Old, the deputy director. He was going to be a scientist, and of course was going into cancer research. When I asked him why, he replied, "Because I like puzzles." The young people coming into science, and the people already there, all want, even need, complexity as their challenge. They all have another trait in common as well: compulsiveness. They are both compulsive and obsessive about their work because the feeling induced by discovery is something that captures and then carries them. The exhilaration takes on the qualities of a "trip"; it is a sensation that must be repeated and repeated. Bob Good spoke of it in these terms: "I remember when it happened to me, when I made my first discovery, and I knew I was somewhere where nobody had ever been before; that I could see and feel something that was absolutely unique, and to have that happen . . . The exhilaration doesn't last for long because pretty soon you are onto the next chase, but it happens frequently enough to become an addicting experience."

Science, then, is a demanding mistress from whose charms scientists never free themselves and never want to free themselves. Their husbands and wives realize this. They may not like it, but they are wise to face up to the reality. Science, thus practiced, can make equally heavy demands on a marriage. For example, Frank, Magda's husband, and Irene, Kingsley's wife, see clearly where they and the family stand in relation to the driving obsession. It can be rewarding, but it also can be stressful and at times thoroughly disconcerting. Because so much of the process of discovery takes place in the streams of the unconscious mind, thoughts can come surging to the surface at singularly inappropriate times. Kingsley spoke of waking up in the middle of the night during that month, with "This new thing with mice going on at me all the time." One scientist has admitted that even while he was making love to his wife, the results of his current experiment would come bubbling up. He loved her very much, and she was extremely attractive, but he couldn't help it. His obsession was such an overpowering one that the mental processes kept fermenting the whole time. Perhaps this explains why, in the history of science, there have been so few examples of great scientists falling passionately and deeply in love, and certainly never to the extent of leaving their science. How many great lovers in literature have been scientists? How many obsessions can a man or woman have?

Within science there is something tremendously deep, driving these people, forcing them to call up new efforts. Even after their discoveries become part of history, become intellectualized, they can recapture the original inspiration and exultation, for the sensations remain. It is just as well, for otherwise the practitioners of science might be tempted to give up. They are doomed to face much frustration. Science is a series of built-in disappointments, so above all, scientists must have the capacity to bounce back, not only at a professional level in the face of their colleagues' criticism, but also in their everyday work in the laboratory. Many ideas which are possibilities, even good possibilities, turn out to be fruitless dead ends. Even the act of exploring these ideas may involve years of technical frustration before an actual experiment can be done. Every now and then, however, something happens which is encouraging, tantalizing and suggestive; then the initial possibility can generate an excitement and motivation which keeps them going over months of routine, irritation, and even sometimes—it must be confessed—downright boredom.

Scientific discovery, then, is a process which is engaged in by as variable a set of people as the rest of mankind. Apart from the fact that they do tend to be something of an intellectual elite, they encompass the whole range of human qualities and political beliefs. They can be nice and compassionate, or they can be mean and Machiavellian. Some believe in God, some are atheists. Some bet on the greyhounds, some play the stock market. Some are devoted to their children, others neglect them. As for compulsion and obsession, these are characteristics that define millionaires, gamblers, artists and athletes equally as well. The distinction lies in the end to which the compulsion is directed, the nature of the rewards the compulsive person can obtain. But looking at all that has been written about science and scientists in the last fifty years, we must admit that there has been a profound misunderstanding, even anxiety, about who they are and what they are doing.

The recommended antidote has more often than not been to emphasize that scientists are human above all. It is salutary to ask why we have needed to do this, and also whether this emphasis on the human aspects of scientists will really meet our anxieties about science. I first came across this antidote in Jacques Barzun's book *Teacher in America*. There Barzun, like so many others before and since, pointed out how sad and dangerous it was that so little of the real nature of science was understood by the general public. He went on to argue that if only we knew more about scientists as human beings, we would come to understand and appreciate their science better. He gave as one of his examples, amongst others, William Harvey. We should realize that he had a very bad temper—had been, in fact, very quick to draw his dagger. Possibly I misunderstood Barzun's point, but I remember being unconvinced by this example from the very beginning. Is one invited to visualize a choleric and testy William Harvey, with dagger drawn, chasing one of his assistants around the room whilst shouting, "I'll make your blood circulate!"? Did his human traits of testiness and irritation contribute to his realization of the closed circulatory system, with blood circulating perpetually in a figure-of-eight motion? I don't know, but I doubt it, for I think the point about the relationship between humans and their ideas is much more subtle and elusive.

In the first place the motives which first drive men into science and then keep them there are extremely variable. Some, like Jacques Loeb, have gone into biology because they wish to disprove the existence of free will; others have entered science because they firmly believed in the existence of God and wished to study his work as manifested in the operations of Nature; others were agnostic. But once a man is within the profession and caught up within the communal enterprise, his personal traits tend to be submerged. This makes it difficult for the outsider to grasp the genuine human elements within science. So we have taken the easy way out and fallen back on the myths: the good and the bad, Sir Galahad with his immaculate concepts or Dr. Strangelove with his Machiavellian obsessions.

So much militates against our proper understanding of science. Its very processes do not help us, and its history, while fascinating, is equally unhelpful. It is a young discipline with limited experience, and compared to history as we think of it, no great sophistication. It has neither its Macaulay, nor its Namier, nor its Isaiah Berlin. The most vivid historians remind us that history is a tapestry formed from individual strands that can be seen every day in the pages of the newspapers and journals, and they have written in depth about the relationship between these individual events and the larger forces that determine the overall sweep of history. But after months of watching the processes of science involving the similar minute day-to-day accretions of detailed knowledge, I concluded that this cannot be done for science. The impulses, feelings and reactions of those scientists I met were part of this knowledge, certainly. Some were caught in the sweep of the larger forces, some in the mesh of small personal impulse. But if fifty years later I had come to read of these days, the personal elements would have totally vanished. Science, as we later read about it, tells us very little about its own history, partly because, as Medawar has pointed out, it embraces it: "A scientist's presence, thoughts and actions are of necessity shaped by what others have done and thought before him; they are the wave front of a continuous secular process in which The Past does not have a dignified independent existence of its own."

Moreover, the established format of a scientist's writing, even if we read it the moment he writes it, helps us very little. It is no good going to *Nature* or reading a scientific paper and hoping to sense the scientific experience. By the time the ideas are expressed, the communal aspects of a scientist's work have been totally drained of their human content.

There are many possible answers to the questions that scientists put to nature. A scientific paper reflects the process of finding the answers, but not the thought processes that led to the framing of the question in the first place nor to the designing of the experiment. This is most unfortunate for us outside of science, since it contributes to its cold image. The format eliminates the excitements, the frustrations, the boredoms and the pleasures—the human experience itself. It eliminates not only all intensely personal emotions, but all communal ones too: whether you do or do not dislike your fellow scientists, think them foolish, stupid, competitive, or just muddle-headed. When I next read in *Nature* a paper by Magda, Kingsley, Jim, or Barney, I will never know the qualities of the life and experience that went into those two thousand words written in terse, indirect language.

Professionally, the scientist must stand aside from everything in his problem except the core of the problem itself. But personally there is really only one thing he must suppress; any tendency to influence the course of events so as to get a result he would like. Otherwise, he is perfectly free to run the gamut of human emotion, and he almost always does. Yet we on the outside have unfortunately come to equate the objectivity of the process with the detachment of the person. Just how deep the gap in our comprehension is was brought home to me most vividly last year, during the time I spent with Jim Trosko. One day I went down to his office to talk. It was two-thirty in the afternoon, and that lunchtime I had attended one of the concerts which from time to time is held in the College of Human Medicine at Michigan State University. On those occasions, nothing else is scheduled, and that particular day we had listened entranced as the pianist swept us through a virtuoso display beginning with Beethoven and ending with Mussorgsky's *Pictures from an Exhibition.* The music expressed the whole range of emotions that I had experienced that morning, so I was in a mood of euphoria as I positively floated down the corridor to find Jim. I went into the laboratory and through to his office. The door was open as usual, and there he was, sitting at his desk, leaning back in his chair and doing nothing. The expression on his face caught my eye, and I said, "Jim, what's wrong? You look very sad." He looked up and nodded. "I am sad. It was the music."

I thought at first he was referring to the capacity of composers to touch deep chords in us all, forcing us to resonate with the whole of human experience, so we can feel extremely sad without being unhappy about any one specific thing. But it was not that. "You see," he went on, "as I was listening, I felt that I could understand, even know exactly, what the composer was saying as he wrote and what he wanted us to feel. But what I know and feel about science is something that I can never get another person to experience, no matter how hard I try."

He was, of course, right. There is an immediacy about a work of art, about painting or a piece of music; the very measure of its greatness lies in this immediacy. In a small measure, we both sense the feelings of the creator and participate in his act of creation. It is quite otherwise with science. No matter what its products—an idea, a mathematical formula, a beautiful suspension bridge or a cure for cancer—the appreciation of the end result in no way opens to us the acts of creation themselves or the processes of discovery or the exultation of the creators. By the very nature of science itself, we are debarred from participating, and the gap is one that will always remain. An analogy can be drawn to a game of chess. Provided you have some skill, expertise and judgment, you can look at a game of chess and appreciate the skill involved and something, too, of the pleasure. But unless you actually are a chess player and can go through the whole process yourself, there will inevitably be a gap in both your appreciation and experience.

The chess analogy is helpful in another respect, too. The moves of chess are easy enough to learn, but one soon comes to see that there are positions in which there always is a right move or a wrong move. If you play the right move, you may win; if you don't, you will lose. Any two good players in any sort of position will play the right move because they *are* good, though their personalities may be totally different. Boris Spassky and Bobby Fischer illustrate this point well. One can go even deeper. Some players will not only see and play the right move, but consistently see and play the brilliant move all the time. Why and how this happens, we don't yet know. We are ignorant of the patterns—cerebral, external and psychological—that precipitate this behavior.

Many scientists, too, are consistently good at discovery; others are not. It is a quality which every scientist recognizes, but which is difficult to describe. It is the same quality that doctors recognize in those practitioners who are superb at diagnosis, compared with those who are just humdrum. These scientists are able to perceive those problems which are ripe for solution, and in this way have already increased their chances for making a discovery. In addition, by some unknown faculty, their imaginative preconception of what the truth may be is always very close to what the truth, in fact, turns out to be. It is as if they have a private hot line to the external world. These are the grandmasters of science, having a maddening brilliance that makes the whole process seem both simple and effortless.

But if there are situations in which there is a right move which any great scientist could in theory make, then where does the uniqueness of the discovery lie? Does this not detract from an individual's personal achievement? This is an especially intriguing question today, since the vast amount of science we are doing makes simultaneous discovery almost inevitable. If Crick and Watson had not put together the pieces of the jigsaw that was the gene, or if Newton had not pieced together the elements of the planetary system, others undoubtedly would have very shortly. The time was ripe and the pieces were at hand. The mark of a man's scientific individuality, his most precious personal possession, lies in the completeness of his solutions, in the breadth of the imagination which enables him to sweep everything up together and bring theory forth. It is the shining "blaze of understanding"—to use Medawar's phrase—conceived and presented in such a way that after the act things are never quite the same again. That imagination is very individual; there is no one type, just as there is no one type of scientist. The enterprise accommodates a whole range of personalities such as those that appear in the pages of this book, or those that appeared in *The Double Helix*, "larger than life, at a strange, contentious, noisy tea-party," as Peter Medawar described them.

If scientists have been encompassed by a myth, society is partly at fault, but the profession cannot escape a degree of blame either. While they actively disavowed the image of Dr. Strangelove, they actively encouraged one of Sir Galahad. As Bob Good once wrote, "From our earliest days . . . we are taught to sing popular songs about science; science is altruistic; progress is facilitated by unreserved sharing . . . Nothing can give a scientist greater pleasure than to see his work as a stepping stone to progress . . . [but] even in our own group one sees, . . .

and from the most effective scientists, evidence of all human frailties . . . jealousy, hostility, selfishness, secretiveness, even surreptitiousness, and prejudice." He draws the analogy with the well-known territorial imperative in animals, the fierce reaction that is evoked "when intellectual territory staked out in relation to a creative experience, an original insight, a chance association, is threatened." It is an excellent comparison, though all too often the profession has denied the existence of the territorial imperative in science. It was Dr. James Watson who really blew the gaff.

We profess to be shocked or disappointed when we find that the scientist has feet of clay; actually, we are perversely delighted. The profession professed to be shocked, too, and it was certainly not at all delighted, for it wanted to preserve the image. When *The Double Helix* was published, it caused a shout of delight from the outside world, matched by an equivalent shout of dismay from within the community. John Maddox, who was editor of *Nature* at the time, recalls how he asked twelve different scientists to review the book, and they all refused. In the end, he had to review it himself. It wasn't that these people didn't recognize the truth in the picture that Watson had etched with a sharp and at times cruel pen, but to show science warts and all, with scientists swayed by competitiveness, sharp practice and arrogance, was in bad taste at its very highest. There was an authoritarian, not-in-front-of-the-children touch about the profession's reactions, a feeling that the realities of professional relationships should perhaps not be admitted; still less should they be so publicly demonstrated to the outside world.

Such reactions are not unique; the screams of pain that arise when one's cherished myths are in danger of being destroyed emanate naturally from all ingroups with large self-interests, as the utterances of the American Medical Association reveal. Recently, excruciating and agonized cries floated up from the Law Society in England when the present commissioner of the Metropolitan Police, Sir Robert Marks, suggested that there might be some lawyers in the profession more interested in themselves than in the practice of law. Professional reactions can sometimes be carried to absurd lengths. I was at a medical conference once at which I quoted a glorious statement taken from *The New York Times*, early in this century, in which Dr. James Walsh argued for the introduction of the horseless carriage on the grounds that it would, "greatly reduce the death-rate in cities." The argument, impeccably scientific, turned on the relationship between the breeding habits of disease-bearing flies and horse manure. Since in retrospect the gentleman's prediction was blatantly wrong, but since he was such a distinguished medical man and therefore could not possibly have been wrong, two equally distinguished but contemporary medical consultants in England were convinced that I had completely missed the point. Dr. Walsh, famous in the annals of physiology, must undoubtedly have had tongue in cheek when he made this famous statement, I was told. But I don't think he was being ironic: I think he was wrong. This sometimes happens. To protest when one's profession is prodded is to fail to acknowledge that the frailty of people and institutions are inevitable elements of any human enterprise.

Emotions run as high, temptations come as strong and weaknesses are as real amongst these people, both collectively and individually, as among the members of any other group, but the point of disagreement has shifted slightly. No one now questions that what James Watson chose to reveal in his scientific "memoirs" was a true statement about scientific affairs as presently practiced. The only question is, Was it always true of science, or are the features of urgency, priority, and competitiveness new on our scene?

Several things are quite unique to science in the last half of the twentieth century, chiefly the extent of science itself and the extent to which it is riding on the back of the taxpayer. When it costs more, both in terms of equipment and because more is being done, when more people are drawn into the orbit and are therefore dependent upon science for their livelihood, the pressures do build up. There is no doubt of the difference in ambience between the American and the European scene. It is possible that America is supporting just about as many scientists as is healthy for the enterprise. The vigorous, intense air of competition leads on the one hand to a blanket approach to science, with everything being tried, but it also leads to pressures which can needle rather than sustain you. Alf Burness was very revealing about this. If asked in England how things were going on, he said, "I would always reply, I am just wriggling along," but in America one says, "Marvellous, just fine." One always says that about one's health, too, even if on the verge of collapse. After giving his very first lecture in America, Alf was told that he had made the wrong response to a question. He had answered, quite honestly, "We do not know." But he soon learned to say, "We are hurrying along with our investigations into just that problem."

This is because everyone wants to get there first, whether it is to the discovery or to the money, so pressures and temptations come at several levels. In order to get funds, one needs to demonstrate results. In order to prove that you have results, you must publish, so pressure tempts you to publish work that is not really ready. In the earlier years of the century, you might have waited. Stuart Marcus confessed to having been absolutely disillusioned with science at the very beginning of his career. Plunged immediately into the pressure cooker atmosphere of scientific research, his first experiences with a whip-cracking egocentric scientific boss of immense prestige—who of course was seeking more—left Stuart distracted and nervous. The pace may also be proceeding too fast for our understanding, since understanding demands reflection. Kingsley and Peter Medawar separately gave me the same scientific beatitude: "Blessed is the man who washes his own glassware at the end of the day, for he has time to think."

In laboratories in America, one moves in an atmosphere of high pressure with no safety valve. Whether one likes it or not, or regrets it or not, the fact remains that a degree of hostility and suspicion is generated that would deeply shock those who still want to imagine science as a kind of intellectual Valhalla, with these knights cooperating for all eternity. Final results may be revealed, but often precious little else is communicated. James Watson was honest about the way in which he acquired the necessary data from Rosalind Franklin, keeping her in a degree of ignorance about the focus of his and Francis Crick's work. Another scientist well known to him is said to have extracted some viruses from a colleague in an extremely ingenious—and perhaps dubious—manner. He wrote asking if he could have a sample of the virus, and having been refused, as his colleague was perfectly entitled to do, he calmly put the letter of refusal into the blender. This spontaneous action was based on the assumption—very sensible, as it turned out—that some of the virus would probably be floating around the man's office, and might well have landed on his notepaper. Is this unfair deception or sheer ingenuity or both?

However, the profession alone has not contributed to these pressures; others have impinged on scientists from the outside. Another new element in the twentieth century is the existence of a vociferous press and a voracious television. The last twenty-five years have witnessed a process of mutual discovery, followed by mutual use and sometimes mutual exploitation. The temptation to announce your method or your discovery or even to flatter your vanity is very real, and one which was not so obvious in the years when the profession was neither big news nor big money. Even that most orthodox of scientific journals, *Nature*, admitted in a recent editorial (March 22, 1974) that science is now show business that "comprises music as well as music-hall, theatre as well as circus." Scientists have been thoroughly ambiguous in their attitudes toward publicity, some honestly eschewing it, others blatantly seeking it, others hovering uncertainly somewhere between, while still others taking the hypocritical stance of affirming their distrust of the media while advancing toward its representatives with open arms.

On the other hand, the press, too, has not always been level-headed. A truthful assessment of any discovery is usually deemed so dull as to not be newsworthy as it stands. Professional pressures on writers and editors to make the news profitable come into play, so the writer may succumb to temptation and seek to make the discovery and the discoverer flamboyant and appealing. Since few journalists take the time, or *can* take the time, to build a realistic picture, another set of images is quickly constructed, distorted by prevailing fashions. So while there are some outstanding examples of superb, balanced science writing, one gets the whole spectrum from the overromanticizing of some undeserving soul and the glorification of a gee-whiz discovery of cosmic significance to detailed relevations of personal vanity and professional villainy. For better and for worse, the atmosphere has changed drastically since the time when the media first discovered science, back in the days of those hero figures Robert Oppenheimer and Jonas Salk.

That the press should report science and scientists in depth is essential. That the scientists should assist in the process is equally essential, for good science writing demands as much research as good science. The old newspaper maxim "Find out what's going on and raise hell" is a valid one, yet one must ask what in science is it honestly fair and right to raise hell—or hopes—about? Equally, the scientific profession has wanted things both ways, the right kind of reporting with the right touch of exaggeration—not enough for distortion, but just enough to maintain the image and bring in the money. The personal details have been fine, too—provided they have been the right ones. "Show us as humans, but not too human" has been their plea. From time to time both sides must step out of the overheated atmosphere of American science and think together of their mutual responsibilities, as they do during the science writers' seminar organized annually by the American Cancer Society.

These morals came very much to the fore in a bizarre episode in which I was unwittingly and closely involved, "The Affair of the Painted Mice," associated with Dr. Bill Summerlin, lately of the Sloan-Kettering Institute. I do not know the whole truth of this matter. The only person who could know that is Bill Summerlin himself, but probably by now he too does not. After seven months all I can do is take my notes, written at the time, and the articles that have been written since, and describe what I saw. I have two preliminary considerations, however. The first concerns the ultimate price that scientists must pay for the privilege of being scientists; the second, the basic ethic to which they subscribe.

Every profession demands a personal price from its practitioners, and science is no exception. Its particular price comes as a result of the communal nature of the enterprise, and because scientists are human they react in very human ways when called on to pay. The price is oblivion. If they do nothing and achieve nothing, they are sunk. If they achieve something, they may still be sunk as far as lasting recognition is concerned. Paul Weiss once said to me, "You know, when I'm dead I will either go up there, or down below, and I will make a point of listening in on all the scientific meetings. One day someone will say, or someone will write, 'Scientific facts have shown that . . .' and I shall purr with satisfaction because I shall know that it was my work that enabled him to say, 'Scientific facts have shown that . . .' And I shan't mind a bit that they don't say it was me who demonstrated that point." He waited for a moment, then turned to me and said, with a most endearing smile, "Who am I kidding?"

It was not that he was a-whoring after a superstar status. Most scientists want something more enduring than a meteor shower. They want scientific immortality, but they know that with few exceptions it is a dream: not only will their personalities be lost, but their work too, for the contributions of the majority, large or small, will be carried away along the flood tide of scientific history. Only a few men like Newton, Einstein, Darwin, Aristotle, and Descartes will survive because of the brilliance of their discoveries and the breadth of their vision. Some will also be remembered because history later proved them wrong, like Lamarck or Lysenko, or because they also became martyrs, like Galileo. But these are the exceptions. The pooling of all ideas is so inevitable that the pride of possession, the struggle for priorities, can be seen in a much more sympathetic light. No scientist ever took the phrase "the disinterested search for truth" to mean that *scientists themselves* were to be disinterested in that search or its outcome, only that they would not allow their own personal feelings and desires to get in the way of finding the truth.

That search for the truth is my second consideration. The basic ethic of science consists of only one rule: it is an attitude to which a scientist subscribes by the very act of joining the profession. It is not necessary to codify it or even swear to it, as doctors have done with the Hippocratic oath, for without it the enterprise could not continue. Bob Good put it to me most aptly, and in view of the episode that was to rock the Sloan-Kettering Institute, his words are poignant: "There is only one basic rule in the game of science, and that is that everyone agrees to work by the rules. You agree to report what you see; you have got to be really honest no matter how prejudiced you are; and you have got to be honest in how you put down the results. There is no other rule at all."

It is because this is the very substance of science that a scientist's honesty is *never* questioned. As the methods have developed over 2,500 years this aspect has become more and more refined. Total honesty in description and reporting underpins a scientist's striving towards understanding of our world. There is plenty of room for dishonesty outside the laboratory, and scientists are no more nor less honest than the rest of us, capable of deceiving their mates as well as the Internal Revenue Service. But the threads of honest procedure and honest reporting stand out like gold in the fabric of the enterprise, and are so ingrained that when the extraordinarily rare cases of dishonesty do emerge they must be seen not as evidence that the emperor has no clothes, but as temporary aberrances, whose basic cause must be found in the clay feet of the people involved.

If total honesty is demanded, what does it entail for the scientist? Again, one thing alone: he must be critical—about other people's ideas, about his own ideas, and most especially about the theories he believes in deeply, the ones that in his heart he wants to be true. These ideas require the most stringent testing of all, and this calls for rigid discipline combined with resilience in order to assimilate the inevitable failures and disappointments which must follow. Of all the professions, science is the most critical. There are full-time critics of music, art, poetry and literature, but there are none of science, for scientists fulfill this role for themselves.

The week of March 25 was my third week at the Sloan-Kettering Institute; I spent it in the Manhattan laboratories on Sixty-eighth Street. Kingsley and Irene were at Canaan and had offered me their apartment, so I had made a whole battery of appointments. I was delighted to find that on Friday evening Sir Peter Medawar was to give a lecture at the Rockefeller University. I planned to attend.

On the evening of March 25, I spent five hours with Bob Good. I had met him off and on the previous week during the visit of the Board of Scientific Consultants, but during that rich, hard-working evening there was enough time to talk in depth about many things: immunology, the general picture for cancer, the methods of science. It was during that session that he spoke of the one "basic rule in the game of science."

Next morning, at ten-thirty or so, I went to the sixth floor of the laboratories, and into the laboratories and office of Dr. Bill Summerlin. I had decided to try and talk with him as far back as January, when I had first heard his name from Dr. Peter Alexander of the Chester Beatty Institute. In that relaxed, unwinding period at the end of a two-hour interview, I had mentioned that my next big stretch of time on this book would be spent at the Sloan-Kettering Institute. We spoke about the place briefly—an institute and director that Peter Alexander clearly admires greatly—and then I finished with my usual question: "Is there anything especially I should look for?" He replied, "Well, there's a man there who claims to do remarkable transplants, but no one else has been able to reproduce his results." He explained something about the work, and as I listened I was moved to comment, "He sounds like an immunological Uri Geller!" Peter Alexander replied, "See what you can make of it. I think you have a very interesting challenge there."

Bill Summerlin was apparently able to get transplants, basically of skin and cornea, to "take" in circumstances where they would normally be rejected. If this were true, his work would have staggering implications both for immunological theory and for therapy. Prevailing immunological theory said that the long-term acceptance of a foreign graft was unlikely, if not impossible, for the grafts would be invaded by lymphocytes and rejection would be provoked in all organ transplants, other than in ones from one's own body or from really close genetic relations, such as twins, siblings or parents. This theory, stemming from the work of Peter Medawar and MacFarlane Burnett, had by then a wealth of empirical evidence to support it, ranging from laboratory studies to surgical experience with organ transplants. Summerlin had challenged the whole effort. His technique was very simple; he maintained the skin in tissue culture for a considerable time beforehand, up to three months, and then used the skin for transplantation.

If the phenomena were absolutely clear-cut, then at least four things would have to happen next: he would have to be able to repeat them, almost on command, whenever he wished, both in patients and in laboratory animals; so, too, would other scientists; there would have to be a whole range of confirming experiments in laboratory animals with different backgrounds and in different environments, so as to exclude all possibilities of genetic relationships; and lastly, someone was going to have to think up a good theoretical explanation to accommodate the new facts which, while therapeutically fantastic, were a total theoretical puzzle, if not a downright embarrassment. I gathered that for all the publicity following the first papers, even the initial phenomenon might just be a passing aberrancy, for in spite of many trials, no one had managed to reproduce the effect.

I met Bill Summerlin in his laboratory and we went immediately into his office to talk. With very few exceptions there is no room for the niceties of furnishing at the institute; the impedimenta of science take priority. His room was the usual small space, with a desk, a bookcase and a small cot. There were cartoons on the wall again, but one was especially unusual, and since I am a Peanuts fan, it caught my eye immediately. It was an original showing Snoopy sitting on the top of his kennel with a look of immense pride and satisfaction on his face. The caption read, "Oh, what lovely research!" In the usual preliminary exchanges before getting down to serious work, I mentioned both the cartoon and the cot. Charles Schulz had been a patient of Summerlin's and had sent the picture to him, I was told. As for the cot, Summerlin often stayed late working in the laboratories, and so slept over instead of returning to his home in Connecticut, as he had in fact done the previous night. He cleared a space for me on his desk, and with charming courtesy, invited me to start. I liked him at once, immensely. There was such an openness and a relaxed ease about him, with no trace of either defensiveness or aggressiveness, that I knew the interview would be easy to conduct and a delight to experience. It was. Dictating my personal impressions immediately after, one of the things I said was, "He strikes me as a diffident, delightful South Carolinian, unusually capable, who is quite candid about his colleagues. He likes working at the Sloan-Kettering Institute, he says, because one has *got* to have candid colleagues."

We began at the beginning. I learned that he was thirty-five years old, born and bred in South Carolina, and that his undergraduate medical studies had been taken at Emory University. He served for two years in the Army's Institute for Surgical Research at Fort Sam Houston, Texas, and in 1967 went to Stanford. He was there four years, eventually becoming chief of dermatology at the Palo Alto Veterans Administration Hospital. In 1971 he moved to Minnesota and worked for a Ph.D. in immunopathology in Bob Good's laboratory. When Bob Good came to the Sloan-Kettering Institute in 1973, Summerlin came, too.

Everyone who subsequently interviewed Dr. Summerlin wrote their own account of the order of his experiments. What follows is the development of his work as he himself told it to me. He spoke of dealing with a very "focused" question which came out of his studies with patients. It arose directly from his clinical experience, and closely paralled, he said, the work of Sir Peter Medawar on burn patients during World War II. When Bill Summerlin was in the Army he saw many patients with mass traumas and became fascinated by the question of what really happens to the body when it loses its skin. Focusing on skin, he became obsessive about it, and a direct sequence of events, which in retrospect seemed to him to be extremely logical, led him to his present situation.

At that time, scientists had no good method for maintaining sheets of skin alive. He realized that it would be very useful to have a skin bank—a deposit of your own skin—so if you experienced burn trauma with skin loss, you could just graft a piece in from your own deposit when required. He started to culture skin but focused his attention on the center of grafts, not the edges. When you begin to culture, the skin is about eight to fifteen cells thick as it is taken from the body, but after a few weeks, the thickness drops down to one or two cells. At this point the skin looks dead and doesn't act like an organ. Bill Summerlin found a very casual experiment done by the famous Alexis Carrel early in this century: he maintained human skin culture for some time in flasks, but concluded that the skin was not viable. To Bill Summerlin, Carrel's photographs of skin cultures looked exactly like his skin cultures, and he believed that the "road was wide open" for him to prove Carrel wrong. This was because he felt all along that the skin *was* alive; there was always some evidence of mitotic activity. He began testing this, taking groups of skin cells from people whose wounds would demand grafts, culturing the skin, and after four weeks or so, bringing it back and sticking it on the wounds. In spite of the reduction in cell depth, the graft would take right off, exploding into a burst of division.

At his skin clinic in Stanford he extended this work, believing now that he had a fascinating problem of biology on his hands. Already the possibility was in his mind that organs could be kept alive for quite a long period of time this way. There was a black man in the clinic who was being treated for third-degree burns on his left flank. Ten percent of the area was burnt. In routine clinical work Summerlin covered the wound area with the man's own skin, and with the patient's permission and cooperation, left four square inches for research purposes. He proposed to grow some of the patient's own cells in culture, let them go down to the apparent dead state, and stick them back into this area in a variety of ways.

The day Summerlin was going to do this, he came to his patient carrying also a dish of white skin from another patient. He said, "I don't really know how to ask you this, but I wonder if you would allow me to put on a bit of this white skin from another patient of mine? I can ask you this, knowing that by all the laws of transplant reaction you will in fact lose it in ten to fourteen days. You won't keep it any longer." The patient agreed, but two weeks later Dr. Summerlin was forced to explain to the black patient why he wasn't losing the piece of white skin, some two inches across and three-fourths inch long. He tried again with a larger piece; there it sat, and it was clear that there it would stay. Completely baffled and thoroughly embarrassed, Dr. Summerlin had the job of trying to explain to his patient that unless they resorted to surgery he was going to have a piece of white skin on his body for the rest of his life. The patient didn't mind; he was routinely discharged from the hospital and Dr. Summerlin was able to keep a close check on him. He examined a piece of the grafted skin under the microscope about a month later, and against all the rules of graft rejection worked out by Medawar and Burnett, there was no infiltration of lymphocytes and no rejection.

He developed this work, extending the tests into other male patients who needed grafts. He now offered them female skin—some of which had been placed in culture, some of which was fresh—as well as using the patient's own skin as a control. The phenomenon, he says, occurred again.

At Minnesota he tried to set up a laboratory model of this culture situation in mice, and there found that organs that had been cultured before transplantation became immunologically neutral tissue. Provided he could find out what was really going on, the possibility arose that scientists could exploit this fact with regard to transplants. Patients would no longer need to be bombarded with those immuno-suppressive drugs which leave them exposed to all sorts of infections. There could be universal organ donors for all transplant experiments, since after culture, all organs from whatever source would be immunologically neutral. He did similar work with corneas from eyes. When corneas are in eye banks, they go very cloudy, but Bill Summerlin told me that he could keep corneas in his culture situation and they stayed quite clear. In fact he began to cross species barriers, something unheard of immunologically, taking human corneas and transplanting them into rabbits. Provided they went through the preliminary culture period, all went well and the foreign corneas were never rejected.

He then told me that no one else had managed to repeat his technique, so since moving to Manhattan, he had begun a penetrating search for two things. First, he wanted to find out what was "going" for him, what was working, so now "they" were preparing an exact manual of their laboratory technique, showing step by step how they were doing this work. Secondly, he began an active search for the mechanism involved, looking at a few of the cells under the electron microscope. The cells looked—according to an electron microscopist, and as Summerlin reported it—like they were "on the launching pad, all primed for vigorous growth." He finally suggested that the mechanism for his phenomena lay in the fact that his cells had perhaps de-differentiated, gone back to a situation in which they took another direction, producing not adult antigens against which the host will react, but possibly those ubiquitous foetal antigens, which, as in foetuses, do not induce a reaction.

We did not talk at length about the precise details of his experiments. Remembering Peter Alexander's challenge, I undoubtedly should have. However, there was plenty of time, for we were going to talk again. What struck me was the scientific uniqueness of this situation: one young man was taking on all the giants—in fact, everyone in the field—and doing work whose implications might bring the pillars of immunology crashing down. I asked him what he felt about this, and he said that the human side of discovery is very disturbing and disrupting, both of the science and of the people concerned in the earlier discoveries. Right now he felt he was in a hurricane with the wind blowing at him from every quarter, and one of the people he was most concerned about was Peter Medawar. Some of the rules which Medawar had laid down were about to be broken. There was nothing romantic about scientific research, Summerlin added. It was tough, hard work, and very rough. He spoke then of the need for candid colleagues, saying that he could never play golf because there was no one to hit the ball back. But he liked tennis because his game was no better than the game of the opponent he played regularly. He needed people who were capable not only of hitting the ball back, but also of telling him where he was wrong.

By the time we finished, it was about 11:45, and we immediately made another date. We would meet that Friday at 3:30 or so, and talk. He wanted to speak with me at length about "discovery," its process, agonies and impacts. Afterwards, we would have an early dinner, then go together to hear Sir Peter Medawar's lecture. As it turned out, he stayed in Connecticut that day and I went to the lecture alone.

For what Dr. Summerlin did not tell me, but what I learned later, much later, was that that very morning he had done something that made my Uri Geller analogy rather more apt than I realized at the time. At seven o'clock he had taken eighteen experimental mice up to Bob Good's offices. The occasion of the visit was to discuss a paper that Drs. Summerlin, Good and Ninnemann were to publish in the journal *Transplantation*. This paper would report the failure of Dr. Ninnemann to repeat Dr. Summerlin's earlier work. The earlier success of the research had been so spectacular that it had received a great deal of publicity—undue and unwarranted publicity, as it now turns out. As Gail McBride wrote in her lengthy account (*Journal of the American Medical Association*, September 9, 1974), a castle of expectation and promise had been rapidly erected on the promise of the Summerlin phenomena and its apparent experimental verification, an edifice to which everyone, the press and the scientists, had contributed. But at some stage one ceases to ride on promise and turns to reality. The work must be repeated before it can be extended, and it must be repeated not only by the original people, but by other scientists. Dr. John Ninnemann came to work in Dr. Summerlin's laboratory; his specific terms of reference were to repeat and confirm the earlier experiments. He could not, nor could anyone else. After some eighteen months he and Dr. Good decided that they had to write the paper admitting this. They asked Dr. Summerlin to be a co-author. This is the usual, honest procedure. Two years ago Dr. Sabin, famous for his polio vaccine, announced the implication of herpes virus in cervical cancer. This, too, received full publicity, which he has never avoided. Recently, he has written a paper—much to the distress of an Italian collaborator, who does not agree—withdrawing his claims for herpes virus and announcing that he cannot repeat his first experiments.

At this time there was a gap of some nine months in Dr. Summerlin's own research work. Between April 1973 and January 1974, the problems of transition from Minnesota to Manhattan—setting up a new department, writing papers and grant applications—had occupied him to the full. Early in 1974, however, he got back to the bench. The mice that he took to Dr. Good on the morning of March 26 were white mice with black grafts which he claimed were "taking," the results of experiments he had set up to demonstrate the phenomenon again. Black grafts onto white mice are more convincing than white onto black, for after the trauma of an operation black skin can lose its pigmentation. The possibility exists, for example, that the white skin permanently in the flank of Dr. Summerlin's patient resulted not from a successful skin graft but because the graft provided a matrix into which the patient's own skin grew, skin from which the pigmentation was permanently lost. There is now some suggestion that the prolonged time in culture makes the skin more suitable to be such a matrix. On the other hand, black skin in a white animal can only have come from a foreign graft.

According to Bill Summerlin's own account, given later in a joint interview to Barbara Culliton of *Science* and Gail McBride of the *Journal of the American Medical Association*, he slept badly, got up early—at 4:00 A.M.—and shaved. At 5:00 A.M., he was drinking champagne and eating crêpes with his colleagues, as part of a surprise breakfast party thrown by his secretaries. Dressings were stripped off thirty mice, and Summerlin selected from these about eighteen to show Bob Good. He said in the interview to the journalists that he was tired, "generally on the verge of collapse," not sleeping well or eating properly, and he was angry, very angry, with Bob Good, who he felt was rejecting him. In any case, in the elevator, he took out his felt tip and "darkened" the graft areas on two of the mice. He emphasized that this was a spur-of-the-moment impulse, in no way premeditated, but he showed the mice to Bob Good as evidence that the grafts were taking successfully. The discussion passed off calmly with Dr. Good glancing cursorily at the mice, but focusing on the paper for *Transplantation*.

Bill Summerlin returned to his laboratory. He reported to his colleagues that Good had said, "Great, great," to the progress of the work, and in spite of the strain and stress, he continued calmly with his work. Midmorning he had the long interview with me. We must have been together about an hour, and it was during that hour that the first representations were made to Dr. Good that Summerlin had misrepresented his data.

One of the laboratory assistants, James Martin, knew every single mouse in that laboratory. He was returning the mice to their cages, and suddenly thought that there were two with black marks he hadn't seen before. He took a swab, moistened it with alcohol, the nearest thing at hand, and found he was wiping off ink. He called Willy Walter, a senior research technician, who rushed down the hall to Dr. Geoffrey O'Neill. He called Dr. John Raaf in the clinic, who came over and decided that Dr. Good must be told. Eventually around 11:00 A.M., Drs. Good and Old learned what had happened. At noon they both saw Dr. Summerlin, and on his admission that he had painted the mice, he was temporarily suspended. He completed his afternoon's work, which included some more experimental grafting and a laboratory meeting. To say that his immediate colleagues were upset is to put it mildly. They were shaken to the core. But even though Dr. Summerlin apologized to his senior staff, he was able to go through the rest of the day, calm and unflappable. One of the senior technicians, angry and disgusted by the whole affair, went home; the secretaries were in a state of shock, as was Dr. Raaf, who could not bring himself to attend the laboratory meeting. The British scientist told me of being angry, desperately angry and sad, remembering how he had come to the States especially on the strength of Summerlin's work to study, and now thinking that this man was playing with all their lives and work. Gradually from the epicenter the shock waves travelled out through the institute and eventually leaked out and into the headlines.

I read the first press reports three weeks later in the *Sunday Times* in England—and gradually over the weeks was sent or accumulated a variety of articles. I learned that a peer review committee had been appointed to investigate the matter, and that their findings were presented at a press conference on May 24. Not only had the two mice been painted, but it appeared that the initial mouse work at Minnesota had been sloppy—the mice not having been tested genetically to see if they were pure strain or hybrids. If the latter, there could well be genetic compatibility—and a graft would be expected to take. Most of the mice were long since dead, but the sole remaining one from Minnesota was tested and was indeed found to be a hybrid between two strains. That it had accepted a graft from another mouse of one of these strains was, then, quite predictable. Other results were hazy and vague: Dr. Summerlin's grant applications carried conflicting statements on such things as the percentage of animals which were successfully grafted. The data on transplants of skin between guinea pigs and pigs to mice were inexact. Worse, the work on corneal transplants in rabbits had been misrepresented on several occasions by Dr. Summerlin, who continued to speak and write of success—as he did to me the morning I interviewed him—when the experiments were, in fact, a failure. He insisted to the journalists that the data had not been accurately transmitted to him, though his colleagues say it was. It may have been a genuine and prolonged error, but in that case he was making claims about a scientific situation whose details he did not have at all clear in his mind.

Many of the press articles came out before the committee's report, and before the long critical study of the whole affair by Gail McBride. Dr. Summerlin himself gave a press conference and radio interview. He said to the press:

> In the light of recent events, no one wishes more than I that the
> actual facts regarding the rabbits were communicated to me. My

error was not in knowingly promulgating false data, but rather in succumbing to extreme pressure placed on me by the institute director to publicize information regarding rabbits, information which I informed him was best known to the opthalmologists, and to an unbearable clinical and experimental load which numbed my better judgment to consult with the opthalmologists, rather than rely on my assumption prior to making any statement.

And so it went on. What struck me was the way in which, in some of the stories, the burden of proof had been so rapidly and neatly shifted onto two other sources, the director of Sloan-Kettering Institute and the pressure-cooker ambience of American science. Personal pressures, lack of proper supervision, undue publicity unsupported by adequate authenticated data were laid at Bob Good's door; indeed, the review committee mildly took him to task for this last point. That these elements were present, no one doubts, but in that case, they have also been present in Bob Good's relationships with all young scientists who have worked with him. The ambience of the American scientific scene, the competitive atmosphere that fosters hostility, exaggeration and secretiveness, is also a real feature in this sad story, but again it is a feature of every scientist's life, though it may press especially hard on young scientists. Stuart Marcus, who had had his own traumatic experiences, spoke of the contemporary concept of scientific "patron"—as distinct from the days of when students were "apprentices." Jealousy and secrecy are such common elements that work is shown only to those who are not feared. A young man with a bright idea, if not already established, must ride on the coattails of a patron, as initially Bill Summerlin rode on the coattails of Bob Good. The patron will help apply for the grant and find the money, using his prestige and connections to see that the application gets consideration. If the young Turk is successful, a patron of sufficient prestige and generous spirit will be delighted, as Bob Good was earlier by Summerlin's apparent success; if he himself is only moderately prestigious, he may react equally kindly. On the other hand he may come to hate both the situation and his protégé and may press hard in a variety of ways on his younger colleague. The struggle for funds exacerbates the role of patronage and, Stuart believes, makes the development of really important programs for cancer much more difficult. But perhaps there is no other way.

Pressures are one thing; honesty in reporting data, another. In science, false reporting is of course self-defeating, since ultimately the results must be repeated. We all regularly deceive ourselves about some things, and can sustain deception indefinitely, but it is not possible to do this in science. Nor do its practitioners ever really want to, for that would be the surest way to end the enterprise. The method has been refined to a high degree of truth; consequently, a man's public statements are accepted as having been honestly arrived at. He may turn out to be wrong, to have made gross errors in technique or interpretation, to have ignored certain critical factors, so while listening to him, others will immediately plan to repeat his work, bringing the full force of their criticism to it. But at the same time, when he says, "This is what I did and this is what I found," he will be believed.

When I reflect now on that delightful interview with a confident and most charming man, who surely has done some superb clinical work in his time, my emotions are somewhat wry. For of course I was conned that morning, beautifully and completely conned, and so, too, were a number of other people. As he spoke, he must have known how tenuous was the fabric of the whole story he was weaving for me. If, as he later insisted, the elements of fatigue, pressure, exhaustion and champagne combined at 7:00 A.M. to induce a moment of aberration, then all I can report was that I saw no traces of this at 11:00 A.M. This is a story of gross self-deception as much as anything else, and a continuous self-deception at that, with a history going back as far as medical school. Gradually a rather different story than Summerlin's emerged as Gail McBride, associate editor of "Medical News" in the *Journal of the American Medical Association, J.A.M.A.*, brought to her investigation of the affair the same critical judgment and resolute scanning of the data that scientists normally bring to each other's work. She traced an insecure and disturbed history featuring another episode of unethical behavior, cheating as a sophomore in medical school (the charges being taken to the school authorities by several of his fellow students), and a consistent looseness, vagueness and imprecision throughout his scientific career.

.   .   .

It began auspiciously enough. As a medical-surgical intern in Galveston, Summerlin was very successful. But at the Institute for Surgical Research at Brooke Army Medical Center he seemed, according to one physician who worked with him, "an immature man who had his difficulties . . . rather mixed up . . . he couldn't seem to adapt and adjust to what was required of him." A number of colleagues felt "that he made the best possible choice when he decided not to go into surgery." So he took a dermatology residency, and later, at Stanford, was "an outstanding resident," according to Dr. Eugene Farber, who is now chief of the Department of Dermatology. Other colleagues speak glowingly of his real interest in the subject and his warm empathy with patients.

Perhaps he should have remained solely in the medical field and in a clinical context, for it was in the scientific arena that discrepancies began to build up. These began at Minnesota when he embarked on the scientific investigations designed to elucidate his clinical findings. One thing consistently impressed me as I stayed with the scientists involved in this work. Though they may be happy to talk generalities from time to time, their daily records are detailed and painfully exact, their protocols minute, pernickety and carefully controlled. The necessity to work to such a regime would drive me insane, but it is vital in science. Apparently Dr. Summerlin did not keep careful records. He seemed "hazy on many details of his work": the review committee that investigated the episode underlined "his lack of properly organized and analyzable data." As for protocol, "apparently none of the mice (at Minnesota) were tested to see if they were hybrids"—and so far as the rabbits with cultured corneal transplants were concerned, Dr. Chester Stock, the head of the review committee, said:

> "When you're a scientist presenting scientific information you should know what you're talking about . . . And he had to admit to us that he didn't know which rabbit was which and yet he was presenting them as if he knew just what had happened with each eye."

According to one scientist:

> "He had inconsistencies in ways to present his own data and in ways to do experiments, which drove some of his colleagues and

fellows mad. When he was working alone at Minnesota, every-thing went well. When he had a huge group, nothing worked; this certainly brings his credibility into question."

Once Summerlin was within the scientific context, however, other pressures encroached, and as Gail McBride reported, a plethora of exaggeration followed.

Dr. Summerlin has also spoken about the pressure of writing articles and grant applications. But according to Dr. Stock: "We have seen many of his lists of publications in which he usually has two pages of manuscripts that are said to be in press or in preparation and many of those are just fantasy . . . Dr. Hadden (one of the committee members) himself went over a list of these manuscripts which were said to be in press or in preparation, and with Dr. Summerlin they agreed that there were only about 2 out of 20 that really meant anything, as far as being actual manuscripts in preparation. The others were just listings of, I suppose, hopes or expectations."

In addition, for the latest edition of *American Men of Science*, Dr. Summerlin listed 12 scientific fields in which he was "expert." Most scientists list two or three. . . .

"In addition," [Joyce U.] Solomon [RN, his former clinical research nurse,] pointed out, ". . . [Dr. Summerlin] told people, such as patients, about specific research projects as though they were in progress, when in fact they didn't exist. For example, he would see patients with vitiligo or herpes infections and give them the impression that several scientists in his laboratory were working hard on their problem and would have possible new treatment available soon. Yet to my knowledge no one in his laboratory was working on either of these projects. These patients received whatever current therapy was available but had high expectations for new treatments or cures due to conversations with Dr. Summerlin. They would call and call to see what progress was being made on the basis of what he told them. Finally, I got tired of answering these phone calls and referred them directly to him. He either would not return the phone calls or would give a superficial explanation that would pacify the patients. He is extremely persuasive and if you don't spend time with him consistently, you tend to believe all his claims. . . .

"Generally, I found him quite disorganized. He didn't seem to know how to follow through, but he could often camouflage it. He didn't shun publicity. We all covered for him because of the way the department functioned.

"Certainly he was under no more pressure than any other doctor at the institute," Ms. Solomon said. "People warned him to get organized."

Pressures were certainly there, but the degree to which they were external rather than self-imposed is a point of contention. For Bill Summerlin saw the situation in a somewhat different light.

"This personal pressure generated by my schedule was aggravated by the professional pressure which is regrettably so much a part of medical research. Time after time, I was called upon to publicize experimental data and to prepare applications for grants from public and private sources. There came a time in the fall of 1973 when I had no new startling discovery, and was brutally told by Dr. Good that I was a failure in producing significant work. (Dr. Good denies this.) Thus, I was placed under extreme pressure to produce.

"Because of these pressures, I became frustrated and distraught, and this culminated in the state of complete mental exhaustion which even the center recognizes as being the only rational explanation for the incidents outlined above."

The picture that emerges from this mosaic shows not a deliberate, cold-blooded Machiavellian deception so much as a sad portrait of a disturbed individual, erratically impelled in a situation which he had neither scientific experience nor psychological strength to sustain.

Maybe the self-deception was not Bill Summerlin's alone, for elements of exaggeration, prejudice and distortion surfaced from all sides as the story unfolded. Somehow the whole episode brought out the worst in a lot of people. As the opportunity occurred to ventilate feelings and dislikes, charity was conspicuously absent. Gail McBride came under pressure—and not from her editor, it may be said—to interview Dr. Good's first wife as if this were either kind, necessary, or really relevant. That most pernicious form of attack, guilt by association, played a role all along, culminating in the words of one critic:

> "The worst, Watergate-like thing is that one of the accomplices in the overall fraud (Dr. Good) selected the peer review committee to investigate, including the most intimate colleague (Dr. Boyce) of his executive vice president (Dr. Old). This is like having Dean and Ehrlichman investigate their own case."

The choice of words, "accomplice" and "overall fraud," for which there never has been one shred of evidence, speaks for itself. Moreover, we not only can imagine, we *know* what happened when Dean and Ehrlichman "investigated" their own cases: the deception was compounded. To equate this with the exact deliberations of a thoroughly stolid peer review committee who knew, as did Dr. Good himself, that the truth *must* come out carries uncomfortable overtones. It was of course the year of Watergate, and this story was suddenly dropped into the maelstrom. In a period during which the press had rightly been acclaimed as heroes for helping to root out vast networks of corruption, it was perhaps inevitable that everyone was infected by the supercharged atmosphere and villains apparently popped up behind every bush.

There are morals to be drawn, of course. Gail McBride drew some of her own that really cannot be improved on:

> But what of the implications for medicine and science? Is this an example of the direction these fields are taking? Is the pressure to obtain scarce grant money as well as recognition—in terms of prizes and awards—so intense that some individuals lose their sense of perspective and others crack? As this case has unfolded, there is some evidence of this. And yet, it seems that the old phrase "hard cases make bad law" more aptly describes the situation.

> If indeed the saga of Bill Summerlin is an exception, making it unrealistic to point a suspicious finger at all scientists, it is time to consider what made it possible. There is first a question that medicine might do well to ponder, and that is whether there is virtue in passing on those unsuited for research or certain medical fields—getting them out of your hair and into someone else's, with the vague hope that they might do better later on, elsewhere—in-

stead of weeding them out early. Many times, those passed on are the unfortunate persons who encounter real trouble in the future.

There is a related point about which to muse, which is that gifted men should not grow so busy that there is not enough time for truly important matters.

Could all this have been avoided? By adequate supervision, could Bob Good have spotted the problems earlier, and is the busy science administrator—a common figure these days—at fault for failing to see what was happening under his very nose? These questions have become more pertinent as two further episodes involving scientific deceptions—one proven, one possible—have surfaced since the Summerlin affair. The man who for many years was one of Dr. J. B. Rhine's closest associates, and who was chosen to succeed him as director of the Rhine Institute for Parapsychological Research at Duke University, North Carolina, was finally shown to have distorted, manipulated and misrepresented his experimental findings over a long period of time. This is a blow which parapsychological research could well have done without, and from which it may never recover.

The second episode concerns forged letters of recommendation written by a Harvard undergraduate, Stephen Rosenfeld, but purported to have come from Assistant Professor David Dressler. These forgeries raise the possibility that the immunological experiments on which the student had been collaborating since June 1973 have been tampered with. Once again, attempts by other scientists to reproduce the results have not been successful. So a statement of "uncertainty and potential retraction" has gone to the two journals where the findings were first reported, *The Proceedings of the National Academy of Sciences* and *Annals of Internal Medicine.* In this case, tampering with the experiments has not been proved, nor can it be proved. Dr. Dressler and another member of the team, Mr. Huntingdon Potter, merely wrote to the journals, as follows.

> Over the last few months we have reported experiments about the existence and nature of "transfer factor." These experiments were performed both independently and jointly over a 10-month period by three people. Our preparation of biologically active material

originally occurred with a success rate of 30 per cent (20 successful preparations). More recently, however, since April, 1974, no member of the group has been able to prepare active material.

This has led us to be concerned that our original positive results may not have been obtained by the procedures described. We leave it to the kindness of our scientific colleagues to accept this statement of uncertainty and potential retraction with our sincere apologies.

Nevertheless, in the case involving an undergraduate student we may assume that there was a significant degree of scientific supervision and yet the possibility of deception still remains. But while for a variety of reasons a number of scientists were prepared to blame Bob Good for the Summerlin affair, alleging that a desire for striking successes diverted his attention from the real facts of the situation, all the statements after this later episode share a real unanimity about the truth of the matter. There is no protection at all against fraud, except the protection inherent in scientific method itself.

Dr. James Watson, who sponsored the Harvard papers for publication, said, "One's mind never considers fraud as a possibility," and in speaking to me, Bob Good said, "I began to have doubts about the experiments, but I never doubted the man." This is always how it has been and how I believe it always should be. In a profession with a clearly understood ethic it is inconceivable that a rational scientist either wants to deceive or can hope to sustain deception. There is no way that a scientist's patron can be protected from deliberate deception short of watching his protégé's every single step, and to supervise to this extent would not only be impractical, it would be unnecessary.

All in all, 1974 proved to be a lively year for the scientific profession. But the epitaph which should serve to lay all three episodes at rest was given by Dr. Konrad Bloch, a Nobel Prize winner and chairman of the Harvard department of biochemistry. "You cannot protect yourself completely . . . any of us could have fallen into the same trap."

The Summerlin affair, deeply tragic for one disturbed individual, is really a footnote to scientific history, as are the other episodes. Personal elements surfacing in a particular sociological context precipitated a professional crisis, but of a moment only. As the bizarre drama ended, "not with a bang but a whimper," and the emotions dampened down, many issues surfaced. The uses and role of the media—publicity in relationship to discovery—may well be central; this is an issue that calls for grave reexamination. Science as it really is, not how society or journalists or scientists would like it to be, must both enter our cultural understanding and be justified. We must ask, then, what it is that we really must know. This calls for reflection, and reflection was conspicuously absent in this episode; it is absent, too, from the pragmatic urgency of the American scientific scene. An atmosphere of calm may be boring to experience, unexciting to read about, but it is nevertheless valuable. If everyone involved in the story had been forced to ponder and weigh, the worst might never have happened.

This, I suspect, may well be one of Bob Good's own conclusions. He admits not only to being sadder and wiser but also to having lost something of his old zest. I am certain, though, that this loss of enthusiasm is likely to be a temporary consequence of a scarring experience and does not extend to a disillusionment with science or young scientists. Otherwise it would be tragic, seeing the remarkable way in which he has always welcomed the young Turks: a competent young man working with Bob Good is neither held back nor put down. But he is making some changes nevertheless. In future, no discoveries will be announced from the Sloan-Kettering Institute until the findings have been independently confirmed by other groups there. The delay won't matter at all: the problems of cancer are not going to be solved overnight, and we in society must be prepared for a continuing commitment.

As for the enterprise, in an ironic way I find it has once again proved itself. It continues to flourish, carried on by human beings who are dead honest so far as the profession's central ethic is concerned. And it flourishes both because of their strengths and in spite of their frailties. I disagreed sharply with H. G. Wells in his cold characterization of cancer workers, but Wells knew how to disarm. From my knowledge of scientific history, both past and very immediate, I know that he was right when he wrote the passage I quoted at the beginning of this chapter: "Science and philosophy elaborate themselves, in spite of all the passions and narrowness of men, in spite of the vanities and weaknesses of their servants, in spite of all the heated disorder of contemporary things? Wasn't it my own phrase to speak of, 'That greater mind' in men, in which we are but moments and transitorily-lit cells?"

The Greeks spoke of it as the god within man.

8

CANCER AND PATIENTS:
BUT SOCRATES HAD HIS FRIENDS

"But surely, Socrates," said Crito, "the sun is still upon the mountains; . . . No need to hurry: there is still plenty of time."

—Plato,
The Last Days of Socrates

CANCER BEGINS AND ENDS with people. In the midst of scientific abstraction it is sometimes possible to forget this one basic fact; yet there is a chain that stretches from scientists with their form of the problem to patients with their form of the problem, and the intermediate links are the doctors and clinicians. With one foot in science and one in the humanities, those middlemen show a side of the two cultures that C. P. Snow never wrote about. Doctors treat diseases, but they also treat people, and this precondition of their professional existence sometimes pulls them in two directions at once.

Intellectually cancer is one of the most fascinating problems; but for the doctor and patient, it is one of the most agonizing. If death means failure, which it should not, then a cancer specialist is constantly faced with the possibility of failure in many of the people he sees. So the dilemmas cancer poses for them are very different in form from those generated on the scientific side.

Now the patients are the reality. The intellectual exercise and the experiments have all been an abstraction, though a very necessary one. This other dimension faces us with equally difficult problems, whose surface we are hardly even beginning to scratch. Again, it was Rachel and Jan, who, by drawing me into their experience, impressed this on me most vividly.

Rachel has acute myeloblastic leukaemia. This is a cancer of one type of white blood cell in the bone marrow. Anyone who wants to know what leukaemia is should read Stewart Alsop's book *Stay of Execution*. This "sort of memoir," as he described it, is a most poignant and revealing account of what it feels like to be a leukaemic patient, and it was a counterpoint to my main theme, the scientific research, for during the winter of 1974 a chapter of it was read every Monday morning over the Michigan State University radio station. One knew, and Stewart Alsop knew also, that the execution could not be indefinitely delayed, though leukaemia is certainly not the immediate death sentence it was ten years ago when remission in leukaemia was a rare event. It was unusual for children to live beyond a couple of years; six months was the most that could be expected for an adult. Now, children go into remission for seven to ten years, and doctors are prolonging life in adults—and a functional life, too. But the first step is to bring the patient into remission. This happens to 90 percent of the children, but to only about 50 percent of the adults. Without remission, a patient will die, and without initial chemotherapy, a patient will not go into remission. However, as Stewart Alsop wrote, chemotherapy, while buying the patient time, "is also a Rubicon." The idea is to knock out the malignant cells, but since chemotherapy can also kill whatever it is in the body that resists these cells, it leaves the patient prone to every possible kind of infection. Thus, leukaemic patients rarely die of cancer. They generally slip away from a severe infection such as pneumonia, or from a total breakdown of the body's functions.

When I first saw Rachel forty-eight hours after her admission, her chemotherapy was just beginning. Eight days later she was in a most serious condition. She had a high fever and a whole battery of infections, with inflammations in the tissues of the leg amongst other things. These probably started from an infection in a minute scratch on the skin, such as we all have from time to time. But because her resistance was so reduced by the drugs, the infection had spread and spread. Internal bleeding extended into her flank; she was coughing up blood, and within two weeks, they were giving her narcotics round the clock. She was slowly dying. It seemed that the drugs were in no way stimulating the remission that everyone had hoped for, and as a by-product, the infections and the haemorrhages were merely bringing her faster towards a death that would have come, with her disease, without treatment. Clinically and therapeutically, she presented a truly horrendous management problem, for nothing could be controlled. The experience and treatment were traumatic and very painful, for Rachel herself, her family and her doctors. The outlook was extremely bad, and one weekend I was told that she would almost certainly die before the next week was out.

I only hoped that somebody was attending to her human needs, which were as great as her clinical ones. I could not get out of my mind the flip reaction of a young intern, a boy from a medical school from another state, who, on one occasion when we were outside the room and he was asked to give his report, said, "Well, we are giving her some antileukaemic therapy and some antiinfection therapy . . . I guess you can say that from time to time we have given her a little bit of antianxiety therapy." One perhaps has no right to judge, but this young man's insensitivity needled me more than anything else had for a very long time. I didn't know whether to be angry with him, however, or with the priorities of the system which had produced him—the word "system" including society as well as the profession. It is always being said that a society gets the politicians it deserves, and I wonder now whether society gets the medicine it asks for. Or, to put it another way, are we right in asking that doctors practice their medicine with humane standards and compassionate morals different from those on which we as a society base our lives? On the other hand, seeing the devotion and personal involvement of Rachel's physicians, I then wondered whether I had been unfair to the intern. Perhaps the flippancy was only his personal camouflage, the way in which he protected his own feelings in a painful situation. So quickly I came to characterize the problem in another way: how does a doctor or a medical student manage to acquire immunity to this constant barrage of trauma, without losing his humanity?

Sir William Osler, the famous Oxford physician and surgeon, did, I feel, a disservice to both doctors and patients, by insisting that the most important characteristic for a doctor was *aequanimitas*, that quality of being undisturbed by good or ill-fortune. An air of balanced self-possession should always be maintained, he argued, so that the doctor himself remains above the human battle, calm and detached, with qualities of judgment and gravity that, godlike, he brings to bear on the patient's problems. But doctors are human, too, and must be permitted to be. Certainly, their agonies are not often revealed, and rarely so at a clinical case conference, but just as there was something exceptional about Rachel, so, too, was there about her case conference, which I was invited to attend. There, the whole history of her disease was examined and discussed by a number of clinicians, and with their help, her two doctors decided how to go on from that point.

For against every expectation she did not die. Six weeks after her admission and some three weeks after her days of crisis, she suddenly went into partial remission. The fever vanished, the infections in her leg, lungs, ovaries and flanks disappeared, and the haemorrhages stopped. Her blood count climbed up and she felt much better. Not unnaturally, she wanted to leave the hospital and go home. Could they let her, however? To a certain extent, the alternatives were limited. They could not, of course, just wave goodbye and forget her. Either she could go and be with her family and wait again for the disease to declare itself, then be readmitted for more chemotherapy, or the doctors could keep her in the hospital and right away begin the second course of chemotherapy, putting her immediately through a physical and mental trial like the one from which she has just emerged.

It was now, for the first time, that I really began to appreciate Dr. Eve Wiltshaw's reminder that with acutely ill patients, we are still working at the frontiers not so much of knowledge as of ignorance. Rachel's doctor, talking to me afterwards, said that he could reconstitute himself from the experiences of his failures only because he wasn't an absolutist. He never really expects that man can accomplish things in a perfect way, and he knows that what he is doing in this sense is extremely imperfect. The kind of tools with which we are now treating acute myeloblastic leukaemia will be regarded with disdain in the future. In a decade or so, doctors may look back on all this as merely one of our primitive first attempts, like the paintings in the caves at Lascaux, where with crude tools ancient man sketched the outline of certain animals. This, Rachel's doctor thinks, is the relative sense with which he can look upon leukaemic treatment. He said, "We are not really treating the disease yet. We are treating merely some of the end stages of the disease. We are trying to push back the neoplastic cells and we don't really yet know what is going on at the point where the patient goes into remission. We assume on the basis of our animal models and other studies that something is happening with the body's ability to recognize cells that are abnormal, but we don't really know. When we do know, and this is the argument for the basic research, then what we do will be less injurious to the patient."

The decision whether to put Rachel back under treatment immediately or to do what she wanted—namely, to be allowed to go home until the disease showed itself again—would have been easy if one could say with certainty just what it was that caused the remission. On the one hand, there was the possibility that the drugs had knocked out the acute leukaemic cells so effectively that the remission was due entirely to the chemotherapy. On the other hand, she may have recovered not because of the drugs directly, but because of herself. Her own response to the infections may have given such a massive jolt to the immune system that it tackled not only the infection, but the cancer cells, too. If this were true, then no one was committed to giving her any more of the extremely painful therapy. An infection would do just as well. Maybe, as one of the doctors put it, more therapy would merely interfere with "the stabilization that she herself and God and Nature had achieved between them." Perhaps on her own she had done a better job than the doctors had done, and perhaps if she were treated again, it would kill her.

The treatments might be still necessary, however. They could help her to survive—but for what, they asked? To go through all that again? If she didn't get severe infections again, it would be possible to keep her going, to prolong her life, but, they asked themselves, what is the price of longevity in this case? The issue they discussed, "quality of life," has no meaning in such a tenuous situation. One could only talk about the quality of Rachel's life if she went into complete remission, and at the time of the discussion, there was no evidence that she would and plenty of evidence that she would not. Essentially, the decisions came down to these questions: should they keep her going with yet another course of chemotherapy, even though it would take her very close to the edge once more? If they did, why would they do this? Would it be because they really believed that what they were doing would prolong her life for a while, though it might at the same time give her physical hell? Or would they keep her going simply because to do so would help both her and her family become better adjusted to her inevitable death? For in their honest professional judgment they knew that they had no treatment that would give her anything approaching a normal life span.

They were between the devil and the deep blue sea, and in many respects, their decision was going to have to be an arbitrary one. This is an essential and recurring ambiguity in much of medicine. There is rarely any absolute, no right and no wrong. One of the doctors turned to me and said, "People say sometimes we have no right to make such decisions. But we have this right and we must make decisions. And we have to make one right now on this patient's behalf." Certainly, with some slow but nonsevere diseases, one can ask patients about the level of ill-health they are prepared to live with, and help them to come to terms with disabilities or defects. In the case of acute myeloblastic leukaemia, however, one cannot ask the patient this question, for one cannot offer them, in all honesty, a life of quality. What kind of life might the patient accept under these circumstances? Whose choice should it be? They didn't feel able to put any of these questions to Rachel because unless she asked, they didn't feel able to admit to her what they knew: that *ultimately* she was certainly going to die from leukaemia.

As I listened, I knew that all these physicians were as deeply moved by her case as I was myself, and this must often be the case, though it is rarely expressed. No one was surprised when her own doctor quietly brought out the core question, making himself and everyone else face the heart-searching issue. When they were unwilling to proceed any further, as they were at this moment, was it because they felt guilty because the treatment nearly did kill her? He said, "We fouled up two weeks of her life. Four patients of mine have died this week and part of me has died with each one of them. I feel guilty and I feel very sad." However, as another doctor gently reminded him, sometimes death is not the worst possible outcome, though this in no way diminishes the grief of the family and the sadness of the doctors. He turned to me with an edge of fatigue in his voice, and said wearily, "You see, we are not experimentalists. We try our best . . . but sometimes we don't know. Just tell people that."

For medicine is not a neat world with neat, tidy problems. One might like to think that there is just one answer: here is a patient with a medical problem; the patient is treated and cured; the patient gets up and goes home. But this is so rare. The beginning of wisdom in medicine, the wisdom that society, as well as doctors, must come to appreciate, is that there is rarely only one answer for any problem, medical or social. There may be possible alternative outcomes, all of which are equally livable. But what so often happens, Rachel's doctor told me, is that many physicians get locked into a way of thought unless they have been educated to recognize and counteract this tendency. "You see the patient; you go through the examination and the deduction; you come to the end and logic suggests a conclusion. Then you think you are home safe and you've nothing more to worry about. But you can't apply tight, neat logic to larger issues, such as the whole context of the patient's problems and the psychological and sociological aspects of his disease. The danger is that physicians sometimes get locked into this situation to the extent of being extremely egotistical about what they are doing and thinking it is right. But falling back upon an attitude which represents security arises out of another problem, for most physicians are constantly humiliated by medicine and the problems it poses, and they react in very different ways. I think if you could make that particular point, it would be important. Physicians are acutely aware of their clay feet, but they try to forget it and deal with it differently. Physicians are human beings, like everybody else, who are trying to cope with difficult problems and who realize that, being imperfect themselves, their solutions, too, may be imperfect."

Then he told me what they had decided about Rachel. They would let her go home, checking in as an outpatient from time to time, and would treat her again later, when the disease declared itself. But he added, "It can be argued, and I can think of some people right now who would say it, that we've done a terrible thing to that woman by not treating her, here and now, at once. What we have done in allowing her to go home is immoral and unethical. You have just seen the conflict, the conflict between the doctor as a man of science, and the doctor as a man of healing, or rather in this case, as a man of 'not healing,' a man whose primary duty is the patient. But in this case, the patient is a sad human being who is going to die. Now, if you like, you can try to reduce every patient to a scientific model, then there's no problem. Or you can let the argument go the other way, and show that too much humanism, too much emotion, too much of a maudlin approach to care prevents 'proper' treatment of the patient. Let's suppose, for the moment, that we knew very precisely what was going on with the cells in her bone marrow right now, in the kinetics of the cell, then our therapy might be very precise, irrespective of what it cost her. But we don't know. It is like going on one of those switchbacks at an amusement park. I know that with regard to the roller coaster which is the progression of leukaemia, this car is going up to the top of the first of the hills. It is in top gear at the moment, going up into a peak of remission. But all of a sudden at the top, I will come to discover just how steep the incline is on the other side. At this point, I have a feeling of anxiety that will hang with me throughout the care of Rachel. For the patient becomes part of one in the process of such therapy, and it is going to be like losing a family member. And, once again, I come to realize that if I cannot cure a patient, then I must help them die."

There is no way of helping anyone die in an objective sense, however, so some doctors do not consider it part of their job. But very early on in his medical career, this man decided that he would never try to isolate himself from the patient and his feelings. There is a heavy price to be paid for this attitude, though he told me that many of the patients help him, too. One patient always sent him flowers, a curious reversal of what normally occurs in hospitals. Another old lady with multiple myeloma, who knew very well where she was in her disease, would always greet him with a smile, "It is a good day, because the sun came up and I am here. Come sit down and talk." The talk would be a kind of two-way therapy, therapy both for the patient and the doctor. I wonder, though, what Sir William Osler would have said?

When one gives a diagnosis with such shattering implications, as in acute leukaemia, generally one of three responses occurs. A patient becomes very upset immediately and begins to fall apart, at which point someone has to help to reconstitute him; he becomes transiently engrossed and depressed; or he becomes very angry with the doctor as the bringer of bad news, the one who, because of his role in making the diagnosis, has "done this to him." Where a strong personal relationship develops, however, there is a great deal each can do for the other, as I was to find later when I talked with Jan.

Though the doctor's internal emotional price may be heavy, Rachel's other primary care physician insisted that not only would it be difficult to be totally objective in critical situations, but it would also be a mistake. At the present stage in our understanding of malignant disease, one is dealing with a natural progression that the doctors try to modify and occasionally do check. So they have a great deal to offer beyond a mere chemotherapy, an approach which, when given alone, Rachel's doctors characterized as a "cook-book approach to cancer." "For otherwise," they said, "you can get so involved in making certain that the data are correct and everything analyzed, that you forget you have a human being sick and dependent on you for certain things." What they would like to set up in these situations is a small unit, a highly trained group of people that are not constantly changing, so that in each eight-hour shift, the same people would come, trained to talk to her with skill, comfort and concern. Then the situation I saw, when as a group we moved out on her, could not in fact occur. This setup, however, requires people who are interested in patients as human beings and not only as cases of acute leukaemia. One doesn't want hysteria, nor an objectivity that can be cold-blooded, nor an emotion that can be overpowering; yet for one of those small instances of time, a patient may need to know that somebody is both sharing the problem and helping. A sensitive group could define a patient's needs very exactly.

At this point I began to see the existence of another source of conflict, a conflict that exists between two groups: the practicing internists, haematologists and oncologists spread out all over the country who are faced with the problem of treating cancer here and now; and those who operate within the context of the three or four specialist centers, such as St. Jude's in Memphis, the Memorial Hospital in New York, and the National Institute of Health Hospital in Bethesda. It is presently an imperfect world, and there are not many places which are both fully equipped and have the expertise to deal with the very complicated protocols demanded by the most up-to-date treatment for leukaemia. Consequently, dilemmas and tensions of another sort are inevitable. I was talking about the problems faced by Rachel and her doctors to a clinician at one of these centers and was immediately met with a forceful reaction: "Doctors in the hinterland have no business to be treating her at all; she ought to be sent to the centers, where there is a leukaemic protocol and a master plan." Another doctor in Michigan reacted sharply, however, saying that such opinions from privileged specialists filled him with an inchoate rage; he felt that it betrayed a great insensitivity to the total dimension of the cancer problem. Generally, there is a real reluctance to send patients away—even if they could all be admitted—and subject them all to those extensive and expensive protocols in a situation where *nothing* can yet be guaranteed. It is hard not to feel that sometimes so much emotional and intellectual commitment is invested in a particular form of solution that an unyielding belief in that solution becomes part of the problem itself. That from the point of view of their leukaemias these patients are best treated in major centers is an assertion over which there may be little debate, but that they should *only* be treated in these places is rather more questionable.

It is well to emphasize how much further we still have to go, even after the intellectual knowledge and a guaranteed therapy are ours. These may be marvellous medical technologies, but in order to have a medical impact, they have to be diffusable; I suspect T. H. Huxley foresaw this. Our treatments must ultimately be both practical and widely available. If all effective protocols can only take place on top of Mount Everest, as it were, then they are no good. Until they are widely available, easily disseminated, easily learned and easily applicable, the quality of the patient's life enters into this equation from the beginning. A patient who, say, is forced to travel regularly from Michigan to Texas in order to receive this up-to-date protocol, with enormous demands made on finances and spirit, may be completely incapacitated for living during that process. The stress on the family—who has to cope with the illness, with the absence, with the strain, and with the financing—may end up being intolerable. The situation is not helped if specialists generate feelings of fury or inadequacy in doctors who *have* to cope with these problems. The social ramifications of cancer, the family problems, the emotions and finances that are involved—all add up to a very upsetting experience. As a society, we are doing very little about this.

Death, so they said, is sometimes not the worst possible outcome. When Jan came to see me, he had realized this. When, I wonder, do we surrender the notion of immortality, yield to the inevitable severing of our hold on life? Perhaps some of us, because of our culture, yield to the fact almost from the moment of birth. Some of us never yield and will fight to the very end. Sometimes, as with Jan, fatigue breaks the will, bringing on what Stewart Alsop described as "a creeping weariness, so deep, that the thought of death loses some of its terrors. Then one will realize that the time has come to die." Yet when this moment comes, what acknowledgement do we want to make ourselves, and what help do we need?

We have not really considered these things, for death is a problem with which we in Western society have completely failed to come to terms. In his book *Death, Grief and Mourning*, Geoffrey Gorer first showed the extent to which we have come to evade everything about death, even the grief and the mourning, embalming it in an aura of unreality and illusion. We are not permitted to die in a manner that necessarily brings ease and comfort to the dying, but in a manner which is acceptable and tolerable to society. As Phillip Aries wrote, "Whatever dignity that remains must be purchased at the price of not troubling the living." Our society does not wish to be embarrassed by unpleasant thoughts, so people who are going to die and those who have suffered loss are socially acceptable only if we treat death as a matter of small consequence, as if it really does not occur. No wonder Jan had to turn to a perfect stranger in order to talk about it.

In May 1973 he was given only three months to live. He came round from the biopsy operation too quickly for his own comfort. He caught sight of the doctors' faces. He had a lymphoma, and three-quarters of his stomach was taken out. After the diagnosis he was admitted to the hospital for radiation treatment—"the frying pan," as he called it—where "they blasted the bejasus out of me." Between May and August, on radiation therapy, he lost seventy pounds, so that by the end of the treatment he was so weak he couldn't even open a door. Then in September, since he was still alive, the chemotherapy began, with a combination of drugs designed to hit out at the cancer, but ones which as usual had side effects. Jan described the process in these terms: "I've been where the kids have gone . . . and I don't like it." For during the first week, in the daytime euphoria fed on euphoria, and at night there were nightmares and madness. He kept extensive notes during this week in the same way that Aldous Huxley did so many years before with mescalin. He hated the mood control, but he said, "When it comes to pain I will take anything. It's the pain I remember."

As Bernie had said to me, it can be a rugged ride, but for survival, there is a great deal that one is willing to bear. Reading Jan's notes, the writing of which must have been its own therapy, it was amazing that this man could recognize and attempt to control both the euphoria and the nightmares.

> . . . A moment of tremendous startlement in the dark, as I tried to orientate myself. I do not know how safe my wife was with me—because for an endless instant, she merged into the night-terror of the beautiful gentle woman, who was doing endless horrors with her unseen hands.

> My nerve endings projected outside my body and I was difficult to be with. This, combined with the sharp pain of an ulcerating mouth, must have augmented the deep depression lasting into the next day.

Such experiences are not unusual with chemical drugs following radiation treatment. Jan emerged from the chemotherapy with his cancer held at bay, and early in 1974 went into the second fourteen-day cycle of treatment. Now there was neither obvious euphoria nor nighttime madness, and though painfully tired, he was able to begin to reorientate himself. I don't think he had read Senator Hubert Humphrey's testimony to the committee hearings on the National Cancer Act, but he acted as if he knew its implications. For Humphrey said, "Time is neutral: it is what we do with it that counts." Jan now began actively thinking of practical ways in which he and society could help others who would have to go through similar experiences; seeing if he could organize discussion groups to cover such problems as medical benefits to the patient and family, the interpretation and enforcement of insurance, ways and means to protect the family and the estate, credit rating and how to deal with medical creditors, and diagnosis—how the patient can help the doctor, where best to go, and how persistent a patient should be. Jan wanted them to know all about facing surgery and just what radiation does and what chemotherapy involves. By making a first step towards helping others, he was trying to come to terms with his own death. Still he had his own individual need which society either did not recognize or did not want to recognize. After four hours I finally turned to him, and said, "Jan, why did you want to see me?" and he answered quite simply, "Because I wanted to talk about dying." "Who is there to talk to?" he asked later. "One must talk about life to the living, so who is there to talk to about death?"

So we talked about it, not only in relationship to Jan, but also with regard to the Turkomans, to all the people I had seen. How different are our attitudes? This is an anthropological question requiring answers that I am not qualified to give, but from what I saw, I conclude that like us, they will prevent death or postpone it if they can. Unlike us, however, they put a premium both on physical risk and upon the capacity to bear pain. They expect to; we will not tolerate it. They respect age and the aged; we tolerate neither. Even when they are old, they know what it is to be a person, but we tend to put people into cold storage even before they are dead. But if we hive off our old people into communities of senior citizens without a function in our society, then what is it that we are trying to keep alive in the Western world? We take away a person's autonomy almost before they are seriously ill, and then in the intensive-care unit, technology removes the last shreds of that autonomy. When we are very old, do we still hold on to the tatters of life, because tatters is all the existence we have been permitted for the last ten years? There is an end for us all, but the Turkomans die in quiet relationship to the cycle of their lives and to the universe. We die aseptically, often away from family and friends, with our sense of personhood undermined, and often undermined long before the threat of death appears.

Some people insist that it will be different. It was different for Stewart Alsop and it will be different with Jan, for both were determined to retain their autonomy. In one of his last articles, Alsop argued from his experiences in the solid tumor ward that "a patient suffering beyond endurance should be given the option of ending his own life, and the means to do so should be supplied on request. An unquestionably terminal patient should be given another option. He should be given as much pain-killing drug as he himself feels he needs."

Jan might well have committed suicide, but he couldn't, because he felt that his family would not be able to bear the experience. One way or another, they had had enough, but he said, "I want to go out well. I want to go out as a person with my autonomy."

Death is built into the biology of our existence even more securely than cancer. It remains a problem for us, not in the sense that cancer is a problem—for we will never cure death, and we probably will cure many cancers. We have not yet come to terms with it in any sense, and even the new surges of concern that there should be "death with dignity" risk substituting a slogan for the solution of a problem. As a society, we are neither prepared to accept death, nor are we prepared to assist those who are ready for it. Somehow we must restore autonomy; we have to permit people the experience of death and share the experience with them, if that is what they want. And for those of us who are left, society must permit us to express grief, for nothing substitutes for sorrow.

We talked for a long time. Just before I left, I told Jan I wanted to give him a copy of my last book, a scientific thriller, which might perhaps divert him for an hour or two. He offered to come with his wife the next morning and take me up to my office, since his wife's office was near mine. I had the book all ready the next morning, and when they picked me up, I handed it straight over. We drove the few miles to my work and said goodbye. Then Jan leaned forward, reached into the glove compartment, retrieved a package, gave it to me with the words "It's for you. I guess it says what I wanted to say" . . . and drove away. I went upstairs and undid the envelope. There was a small book inside, inscribed "From a friend, to a friend." The book was *The Last Days of Socrates.*

But Socrates had his friends with him when he died.

If I was consistently reminded that death is not the worst possible alternative, I have also just been reminded that death is not the only alternative. When I first wrote this chapter, it was seven months since I had seen Rachel or Jan, and I had just received a letter from the haematologist who had been treating them both. He wrote, "You will be delighted to know that both Rachel and Jan are well into good remissions. Rachel has gone off on vacation with her husband and family and Jan is very active. They are both coping well."

By the time I returned, however, ten months later, Rachel's condition was serious. She had relapsed and was back in the hospital. She had never really achieved a complete remission and was now caught on the roller coaster of illness, improvement, then illness again. I saw her regularly during this period right up to the moment she died.

I also saw Jan. He came over to the house and we went for a walk in the autumn sunshine. I didn't recognize him: well, buoyant, he literally hauled me over a seven-foot metal gate on our way to the river. Ebullient, vibrantly alive, he was laughing as he said, "I never expected to see you again. I thought I'd be dead."

EPILOGUE:

SQUARING THE CIRCLE

IT IS NOW well over a year since I began this work, and during that time one person at least moved back onto the human stage. Caught up, as I was, by this human action, I can never withdraw. For all of us—doctors, scientists, Rachel, Jan, the Turkomans—everything is not "quite the same moment of time."

Why am I so positive, given that I believe we will never totally eradicate cancer? It is because I see from the work of all these remarkable people, spread all over the world, the possibility that within five or ten years we will be raising our level of understanding to a new and infinitely more acceptable plane. We could even now, if we chose, *avoid some 60 percent of all cancers* by prevention at a personal and industrial level, and why as a society we fail to do so is a fact which consistently baffles, distresses and finally defeats me.

Be that as it may, we shall soon begin to identify cancer earlier by using new techniques of diagnosis. With increasingly sophisticated tools, both chemical and immunological, we shall be able to improve therapeutic methods faster and more effectively. With the new theoretical understanding of cancer that is sure to come, we will be able to increase our capacity to deal with cancer effectively, even though we may never conquer it absolutely.

Most scientists have been frank about this last point. Rensselaer van Potter, from the McArdle Cancer Institute in Wisconsin, recently said at a conference in Japan, "I must caution you that understanding is not synonymous with conquering the disease. I do not believe that such a goal is realistic, although we must continue to work for maximum results. What we can look forward to on the basis of better understanding is an increased ability to prevent cancer, to evaluate the genetic and environmental components of the disease, and finally to treat various special manifestations of the disease."

At the same time, we shall also be learning to cope with the disease psychologically, both as individuals and society. It is already clear that rational acceptance of cancer as a human disease is preceding rational understanding of cancer as an intellectual problem. During the preparation of this book, Betty Ford and Happy Rockefeller had their operations under the full scrutiny of the public. Since then, as a new, realistic dimension has entered into our attitudes, more has been written and openly discussed than ever before. At the end of the work, I asked Bob Good, present director of the Sloan-Kettering Institute, and Sir Alexander Haddow, past director of the Chester Beatty Institute of London, how they felt. What were their rational expectations? What would they like to say to the wider public? Bob hesitated for a moment, took a deep breath, smiled, and then spoke in his characteristic large way, with his resonant Midwestern voice: "Just keep the faith, baby. Give us time." The breadth of his apartment in New York, with its glorious views, contrasted sharply with the small room in Surrey where I was to sit opposite Alex Haddow. The message was very much the same, though. I was greatly moved by this brilliant man, now blind, staring unseeingly at me across the desk. "What's it really like?" I asked him. "Just how would you characterize cancer?" He answered in a quiet, clipped Scottish accent: "I have always spoken of it as 'squaring the circle.' Cancer is such a naturally occurring event that in order to cure it, you have got to make everything go backwards. We have to go against the natural grain, and when we do it, we will have squared the circle."

I pressed him, "If it is as difficult as all that, why are you so sure that we can do it? Squaring a circle is generally considered an impossibility, anyway. So how can you be so certain?"

Alex Haddow too waited a moment, then smiled and said quietly, "Och, well, you see, because Nature does it herself sometimes."

Nature does it herself sometimes, so eventually we shall, too. This is a fundamental tenet of scientific faith, that with minds and methods we can reach out and come to understand the natural processes occurring in the world. There will be no miracles, and we would be foolish to expect them. Some may ask, as the young American in Tehran asked me, why bother? seeing that we guarantee neither total eradication nor total cure. And even if we did find a cure, the increase in life expectancy would be minute. The vast sums of money that would be required are, on the face of it, out of all proportion to the statistic: given no more cancer, the average increase in life expectancy at the age of seventy would still be only about 1.5 years. So what is the rationale, the American asked me, if the end result is so minuscule? To pose the question in such cold-blooded terms is once again to ignore that haunting dimension of cancer—the human being. Sometimes arguments have to be made on compassion and compassion alone, not statistics or cost benefits. Knowledge and understanding in medicine must be directed toward the elimination of those conditions, medical and social, which are agonizing for people at any stage.

If cancer will never be totally eradicated, however, are people going to feel betrayed? As oversell breeds more disillusionment, is my Rye taxi driver going to be mad as hell at having been presented with yet another unfulfilled promise? Is the backlash that John Maddox predicted in *Nature* going to be severe? I hope not. Our efforts *are* justified, though I could not honestly blame people for doubting this; at times I, too, have been tempted to cynicism by the public relations sell on the promise of cancer research. As a member of society, however, I think that a feeling of betrayal can never follow a realistic assessment and rational expectations. Betrayal will come, though, if once having solved the scientific problem as effectively as we can, we suddenly stop there and call off all further effort and money. If all our sophisticated methods of prevention and therapy are not finally made widely available, disseminated to the Turkomans and to the poor with the same concern and compassion that scientists now bring to the problem itself, then one can talk of betrayal. The poor are paying for the research with their taxes, just as much as the rich with theirs. If the cost-benefit argument is not applied to the basic research, then why should it be permitted to apply to the transmission and spread of the therapy? I want the Rye taxi driver to be able to go for treatment without having to travel a thousand miles, and without having to burden himself and his family financially. The costs can be staggering: $60,000 was the sum total involved in Rachel's care. Unless our collective social conscience says otherwise, the treatments may still remain selective.

I am finally reminded, once more, of my colleague's injunction, "You must not think you can play God; in this business it is enough just to be human." As this task nears its end, I have an acute sensitivity to the remaining gaps. There are so many: between the scientific community and the public at large—for in spite of all that has been said and written, the level of mutual misunderstanding is still very great; between the profession of medicine and the public and between the clinicians and scientists. These gaps are nothing, however, compared with the one I see which separates our intellectual activities as human beings from our compassionate acts. Intellect without compassion is nothing; compassion without rationality is futile. As a society, we have considerable intellectual and technical resources, but it is that universal compassion we are lacking, a lack generated from degrees of insensitivity even as we preach understanding. It is so easy to say that if people really only understood cancer, they could be totally rational about it. All the things we are advised to do are true: to look for early warnings, to see the doctor early, to avoid certain practices. Yet since we are human beings, we are not always rational beings, especially when pain is involved. Indeed, it is irrational to expect us to *be* rational about painful disease and illness. Those who work on the various dimensions of cancer realize that they will always have to take care of human fears and human irrationalities; therefore, as our knowledge grows, we are justified in expecting society to develop more humane attitudes towards those with cancer.

For too many unhappy attitudes still persist, hangovers from the earlier years, attitudes which are neither expected nor bargained for. A mastectomy is bad enough without any additional burden. On March 2, 1974, *The New York Times* ran an article about the difficulty experienced by "cured" or "symptom-free" cancer patients in finding jobs, and even now, Jan tells me that as he seeks a job again, he and his colleagues must constantly skirt around the issue of his illness. There are between 1.5 and 2 million like Jan in America, and this number will continue to grow as our treatments get more and more successful. Society still reacts with insensitive superstition to people who have had the disease, and this is one of the most important human dimensions of all that we must now confront.

On the other hand, we *can* live with human fears as well as with successes, and some agonies will always be there. If cancer is one price we pay for life, then knowledge of our own mortality is one price we pay for consciousness. Grief too is a price that must be paid for our human loves.

Better this than to be a stone.

> "Far better 'tis to die
> the death that flashes gladness,
> than alone, in frigid dignity.
> To live on high.
> Better, in burning sacrifice
> be thrown against the world
> to perish, than the sky
> to circle endlessly
> a barren stone."
> —Anonymous, *Nature*, August 26, 1933.

GLOSSARY

Cancer: I can only say I wish we really knew. It is like St. Augustine's definition of time: "If no one asks me I know well what time is; if anyone asks me I know not." We all know what cancer is at the level of the patient. We don't yet know what cancer really is at the level of the cell.

Carcinogenesis: This is simply the process whereby normal cells are converted into malignant cells; carcinogens are the material that induce this process.

Clone: This is just another word for a "colony"; we talk about a cancer cell dividing rapidly and forming a "clone." This merely means that it has divided and from the original cell a colony of similar transformed cells has formed.

Metastasis: This word has both Greek and Latin origins. *Meta* means change of place or condition or nature; *stasis,* standing. In cancer, *metastasis* refers to a cell which has slipped out of the colony, which was perhaps a tumor, and now wanders around the body. It is carried via the blood vessels, and eventually settles down and forms a secondary tumor at a new site. It represents the most lethal problem in cancer.

Genetics: The science that deals with heredity and tells us why we are or are not like our parents. In every cell in the body there is a *nucleus;* in the nucleus are threads, the *chromosomes;* along the chromosomes are the *genes.* These are specific and complicated molecules whose structure was first worked out by Crick and Watson. They are made of two forms of nucleic acid, DNA and RNA.

DNA: This is the fundamental *nucleic acid,* whose properties are described in Chapter 3. It gives the blueprints to the cell for making proteins.

Proteins: These are extremely complicated molecules whose structure determines the specific functions of a cell. So muscle cells have one form of protein, nerve cells have another form. The process of getting from the nucleic acid—DNA—to a protein, is mediated by another nucleic acid, RNA.

RNA: This is a second form of nucleic acid, slightly but vitally different in structure from that found in the gene. It is not contained within the nucleus, but moves between it and the site in the cell where proteins are made. The whole process is mediated by enzymes.

Enzymes: All living processes are essentially chemical reactions, which can be slowed down or hurried up by enzymes. Enzymes are nothing more than biological catalysts—that is, they are substances produced by the cell which speed up or affect these living processes, but which themselves are not changed at all.

Antibodies: Those substances, proteins, which appear in the blood and are produced by the body in response to foreign substances or antigens.

Antigens: This is a general term for any foreign material—for example, a virus or a bacterium or any substance injected into the body. To increase the "antigenicity" of something means to increase in some way its "foreignness" to the body. The immune response is due partly to the activity of lymphocytes.

Lymphocytes: These are a form of white blood cell; they originate in the lymphoid tissues of the body.

E. coli: A small bacterium, normally in people's intestines, where it lives undisturbed. It is a scientific "war-horse" in that it was by experiments on *E. coli* that so much of our understanding of molecular biology has come.

ABOUT THE AUTHOR

JUNE GOODFIELD was initially trained as a zoologist. After a year's research at Oxford, she took her doctorate of science in the history and philosophy of science at the University of London. For the past twenty years, she has been actively concerned with the interface between science and society, and with the relationship between individual scientists and the ideas they hold. She is currently a visiting professor in medicine and philosophy at Michigan State University, and has taught at Harvard, Wellesley, and the University of Leeds. While serving as Assistant Director of the Nuffield Foundation in London, she produced and directed a number of documentary films on science, one of which won the Bronze Medal at the Venice Film Festival, and also co-wrote three books on the wider dimensions of science, *The Fabric of the Heavens* (1962), *The Architecture of Matter* (1964), and *The Discovery of Time* (1965). She is also the author of the scientific thriller *Courier to Peking* (1972). A Fellow of the Royal Society of Medicine, June Goodfield recently served as consultant to the Iranian government for their paramedical program, and when not in residence in Michigan, lives in Europe.